BREATHING

BREATHING

An
Inspired
History

Edgar Williams

REAKTION BOOKS

To my brothers, Derek and Steven

Published by Reaktion Books Ltd
Unit 32, Waterside
44–48 Wharf Road
London N1 7UX, UK
www.reaktionbooks.co.uk

First published 2021
Copyright © Edgar Williams 2021

Printed and bound in Great Britain by
TJ Books Ltd, Padstow, Cornwall

A catalogue record for this book is available from the British Library

ISBN 978 1 78914 362 1

CONTENTS

PREFACE

The biology of breathing has been a lifelong fascination of mine. It is a phenomenon I have spent my career studying in creatures of all sizes, from small aquatic crustaceans to fish and humans. Along the way I have read widely on the subject, its history and its background, not only to inform my own research but that of students to whom I have had the great pleasure of teaching respiratory physiology for many years. As a respiratory physiologist investigating the mechanisms of breathing, I have travelled the world working in the very laboratories where many of the great discoveries in the science and history of breathing were made. In any series of lectures on the physiology and pathology of breathing, the names of the scientists and physicians who first made these discoveries arise, since they often named the mechanisms they had discovered after themselves: hence we have the Bohr effect, Cheyne-Stokes breathing and Guillain-Barré Syndrome, to name but a few. Research into the cause and management of respiratory illness is important, as it remains one of the greatest causes of global morbidity and mortality, affecting young and old alike.

The history of how we gained our present understanding of breathing is both long and fascinating. It spans many centuries, progressing in fits and starts as major discoveries suddenly revealed new insights into the mechanisms of breathing, such as the first microscopic examination of the lungs by the anatomist Marcello Malpighi (1628–1694), the discovery of oxygen in the eighteenth century, and the identification of the tuberculosis bacterium by Robert Koch in 1882. Historical epidemics of polio, tuberculosis and influenza have shown us how important breathing is to our health. The twentieth century brought huge increases in chronic incurable respiratory conditions such as asthma and smoking-induced chronic obstructive pulmonary disease (COPD). In the twenty-first century, methods of improving health and wellness, such as yoga and meditation, have been popularized. Central to their practice is the self-control of breathing, which helps to manage stress and ease the pressures experienced in everyday life.

Recently air pollution has focused the health-conscious public and governments of the world on the long-term impact of our health. Researchers have realized that ultra-small carbon particles from vehicle exhausts can enter the blood via the lungs and lodge in tissues within the brain and heart. Breathing has gained new cultural relevance with the emergence of the world-wide Covid-19 pandemic in 2020. The unknown virus, which originated in China and is new to the human species, spread rapidly around the world, infecting and killing millions of people. This coronavirus enters bodies through the delicate respiratory membranes in the lungs. On its arrival, suddenly breathing other people's breath became potentially dangerous to life, as nobody had any immunity to the virus (officially named SARS-COV-2). Quarantine, isolation and physical distancing became global watchwords as every country's economy shut down in an attempt to keep everyone safe. We all had to breathe within our own individual space, as did our nearest and dearest.

In most cases of Covid-19, the disease caused by the virus, the viral infection causes mild symptoms such as persistent coughing, a raised body temperature and aching limbs. Most people who catch the virus experience these mild symptoms, which pass quickly, but in a few cases, particularly vulnerable members of the public such as the elderly and those with heart disease, virus-induced pneumonia develops, making breathing difficult. Indeed, staying alive depends on breathing supplying the body with enough oxygen. Many of those who recover in full have commented on their struggle to breathe and how frightening this sensation can be. For the unfortunate few whose bodies over-react to the infection, in whom a 'cytokine storm' develops into pneumonia, the only solution is mechanical ventilation and seda-tion until the storm is over. This book describes how, through the development of our understanding of breathing, we conceived the technology to support breathing, whether it be partially via a mask or fully by ventilator. It tells the story of how physicians and scientists sought to eliminate respiratory illness, and how they not only discovered the secrets of breathing but developed machines to support it. The innovations have helped to prolong life, and aid breathing on mountain tops or when diving beneath the sea.

Throughout, I have sought to answer a single question: why do we breathe the way we do? This book sets out the evidence.

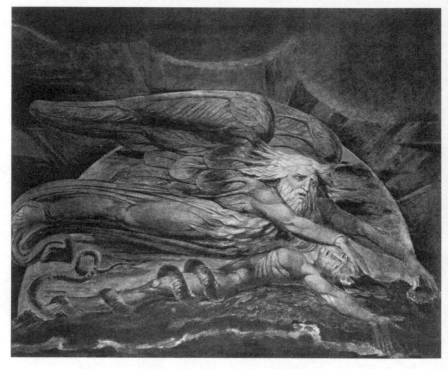

William Blake, *Elohim Creating Adam*, 1795, ink and watercolour on paper. God creates Adam from dust; man is dragged from the spirtual realm and made material.

ONE

THE BREATH OF LIFE

B reathing is life. Day in and day out, with little thought, we quietly breathe to and fro, our chests rhythmically expanding and falling. Drawing breath is one of the first and last things we do; it is influenced by our emotions, behaviour and activity. Often we notice a change in breathing only during periods of ill health. Respiratory diseases, whether the common cold or asthma, make breathing harder. Breathing permeates our culture and is part of the human experience. Many of our greatest scientists and intellectuals have contributed to our understanding of this simple but complex process. Since Neolithic times the act of breathing has provided a spiritual link to the mystery of life.

Breathing is automatic; we inhale and exhale, *ad mortem*. Nowadays we all know the purpose of breathing: as young children we are told that breathing fulfils our requirement for 'air'. Only later, as our education progresses, do we discover that this 'air' is oxygen, the essential gas that keeps us alive and vital. Finally, we learn of breathing's dark side: the 'evil' carbon dioxide, a toxic by-product of cellular metabolism, a gas poisonous to our cells, a gas we must constantly expel to stay alive. While the ancients understood that we need to breathe, they had no idea why. The concepts of air and gas were unknown to them and the anatomy and physiology of lungs were a mystery. Without modern understanding, breathing was considered a spiritual process, connected with the vital forces of life.

The quest to understand breathing has played a large part in human culture and history. Breathing has been central in the development of many of the world's religions and philosophies, and to the understanding of our physical and chemical environments. It has stimulated industry, invention, innovation and imagination.

Early Breathing

Breathing has played a pivotal role in our evolution. Over time it has allowed the development of subtle differences and changes in the stature and function of our ancestors, including our distant, now-extinct human relatives such as the Neanderthals and Denisovans. Altering the way we breathe has allowed our society to develop agriculture and industry. Respiration, the act of breathing, is mentioned in the earliest written histories, with the Greeks being among the first to question its purpose. For these early civilizations, breathing was an ethereal and spiritual phenomenon. It stood for a force of nature or represented God; it was a presence, an embodiment of the Holy Spirit. In the Christian Bible, in Genesis, which marks the beginning of human consciousness, God provides humans with breath as a climax to the formation of the universe and earth. Genesis states that on the sixth day of creation, God created humankind: He 'formed the man from the dust of the ground and breathed into his nostrils the breath of life, and the man became a living being' (Genesis 2:7). Thus Adam was born. Many centuries later, this divine association was expressed by the scientist Charles Darwin in the closing paragraph of his famous book on evolution, *On the Origin of Species by Means of Natural Selection* (1859):

There is grandeur in this view of life, with its several powers, having been originally breathed by the Creator into a few forms or into one; and that, whilst this planet has gone circling on according to the fixed law of gravity, from so simple a beginning endless forms most beautiful and most wonderful have been, and are being evolved.

For millennia, the belief in the spiritual role of breathing persisted. The first to expand on this spiritual role were the Greeks, who postulated that breathing supplied a substance called pneuma, the spiritual essence of life. This concept lasted into the sixteenth century. The medieval period saw the appearance of the first pharmacopoeia, or herbals, which provide intricate descriptions of concoctions and potions to treat respiratory disorders such as colds, asthma and tuberculosis. At first the active ingredients came from common indigenous plants but, with global exploration, they came increasingly to Europe from Asia and the New World. When these were combined with new chemical methods, the first man-made medicines were created. Although primitive, these new medicines gradually led to the view that breathing had an organic basis, supporting the idea that disease was caused by an imbalance of the humours.

At the beginning of the Renaissance in fifteenth-century Europe, human anatomists such as Leonardo da Vinci began to explore the body in greater detail and note the structure of the lungs. These intricate observations suggested to anatomists that the lungs had been 'designed' for a purpose beyond the containment of pneuma. The mechanistic view of breathing was born. At first only the lung's gross anatomy was defined, but after the invention of the microscope in the late sixteenth century, the Italian Marcello Malpighi became the first to observe and describe the minute structure of the lungs, albeit in frogs, describing for the first time the true functional unit of the lungs, the alveolus. It is this small bag-like structure wherein gas exchange takes place, where oxygen enters the blood and carbon dioxide moves in the opposite direction, from the blood into the air filling the alveoli. Parallel to these discoveries were great advances in the understanding of the physics and chemistry of air. The relationship between pressure and volume began to be elucidated, leading to further experimentation that showed 'air' existed in many forms and was not a single ubiquitous entity but consisted of mixtures of gases. This was a huge conceptual leap forward in our comprehension of the world. Eventually these mixtures were reduced to their elemental and chemical forms, with the discovery of gases such as nitrogen, oxygen and carbon dioxide. With the dawning of the Victorian age and the industrialization of society, the finer details of how breathing works began to be elucidated as improvements in technology allowed the construction of better scientific instruments. The age of the professional scientist began, first in Europe, for example in Germany and Denmark, then in Scotland and finally in England. The final great breakthroughs came in the twentieth century with the two world wars, both of which instigated tremendous advances in technological industries such as aviation, diving and space travel.

Breathing-associated diseases have been a constant companion of humankind throughout our history and have taken many centuries to understand. As factual discoveries on the anatomy, biology and chemistry of breathing progressed and multiplied, this knowledge was applied to understanding the pathology of disease, whether acute or chronic, whether infectious or forming spontaneously, such as asthma. With the discovery of germs, bacteria and viruses came the realization that airborne disease was not transmitted by miasmas and ephemeral spirits. With industrialization came air pollution, and it soon became clear that breathing clean air was important in maintaining good personal and public health. The history of how these discoveries were made show how serendipity, and sometimes genius, contribute to today's environment and culture, which are still blighted by air pollution and iatrogenic or man-made respiratory disease.

The Evolution of Breathing

Active breathing common among animals of all sizes, be it fish, bird or mammal, including ourselves. It is easy to observe, this physical and mechanical process that requires specialized organs such as lungs or gills, however primitive. Slugs and snails breathe via the pneumostome, a flap that slowly opens and closes once or twice a minute, each time trapping air inside a single lung, a moist empty space. Frogs are well known for gulping air and expanding their cheek pouches while breathing. In humans, breathing can easily be observed as the chest rises and falls. The act of breathing is a vital life-giving process and its evolution stretches back many hundreds of millions of years to the Cambrian period at the beginning of the Phanerozoic era (around 600 million years ago), when the first multicellular organisms evolved. Before breathing could evolve, a breathable atmosphere was required. There was little oxygen in the early Earth's atmosphere, and the first rise in the atmospheric oxygen levels occurred during the so-called Great Oxygenation Event (GOE) at the beginning of the Proterozoic era, 2,500 million years ago. A second event occurred later, during the Phanerozoic era, when atmospheric oxygen levels settled at the 21 per cent we know today.[1]

Breathing did not begin with the medium of air but with water, with which the first shrimp-like creatures ventilated their gills. The advantage of actively directing a flow of water over primitive gills is that it allows the dissolved oxygen in the water to be extracted in larger quantities than the passive uptake of oxygen

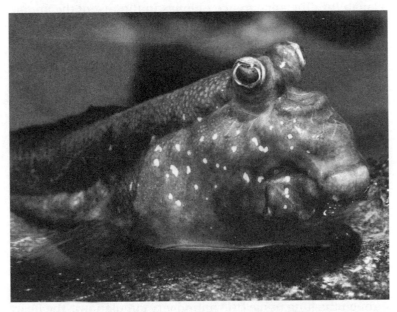

The mudskipper (*Periophthalmus barbarus*) breathes by filling up its mouth and gill cavity with moist air. Its gills are unsuitable for breathing when submerged in water and the fish will drown if placed in deep water.

by diffusion alone. This breathing method gave these creatures more energy, allowing them to grow bigger and faster than their passive-breathing contemporaries. Around 400 million years ago, ancient fish took the evolution of the gill further when a few species began to leave the water and breathe air instead. At first they became partial air breathers, moving between the air and water, finally evolving into full air breathers and leaving the aquatic environment behind. Further evolution led to the amphibians, reptiles, birds and mammals we know today, all of whom use lungs to breathe.[2]

Insects breathe through a system of tubes and, like animals, rely on aerobic respiration (they consume oxygen). These tubes are largely static, though they do exhibit very slight mechanical breathing movements, so air must diffuse into the body directly from the atmosphere. Diffusion is not very efficient beyond a distance of a few centimetres. This is one of the reasons why insects are limited in size, as increasing size increases the demand for oxygen as well as the diffusion distance, which reduces oxygen availability. The appearance of lungs in the rest of the animal kingdom, with their ability to move air tidally back and forth over relatively large distances, overcame the limits of diffusion and appeared early in the evolutionary process; thus tidal breathing is common today in humans and most other terrestrial animals.

Breathing in Utero and Beyond

At birth, one of the very first things we must do is to take a breath. We gasp and breathe; often we bawl and cry. Air floods into our now-inflated lungs and our lifelong dependence on it begins. Once the umbilical cord is cut, the last physical link with the mother is severed and oxygenated blood now must be renewed by passing through the new lungs. Immediately after birth the blood is rerouted around the body and passes for the first time through the lung tissue (the pulmonary circulation). The heart and lungs work together until death, the heart beating around five times for every single breath.

Around eighteen days after conception, when the egg and sperm have met in the womb, the resulting embryo develops its first organ, the heart, and the associated cardiovascular system; this system is essential, providing the means for oxygen, nutrients and growth factors to be rapidly and thoroughly circulated around every developing cell and tissue. However, the lungs are less developed; their rate of growth is more leisurely, as the lungs are not needed during the forty weeks of gestation in the womb. The growing foetus still needs plenty of oxygen, but this is all supplied by the mother via the placenta, which acts as a surrogate lung and liver. In the placenta, oxygen and carbon dioxide exchange occur between the foetal and maternal blood.[3]

In the foetus the lungs begin forming after five weeks, developing first as a bud (called the respiratory diverticulum) on the developing foregut. This grows forwards and develops a small trachea (the windpipe), and then splits into the two lungs, left and right. The point at which the trachea is joined to the primitive gut later becomes the junction between the oesophagus, larynx and pharynx. In the small lungs the two primitive airways elongate and continue dividing throughout gestation, so one trachea leads into the thousands of small tubes found in the mature lungs. After 24 weeks of growth these airways eventually terminate in millions of alveoli. Although the lungs are not yet fully functional, they can be used if the baby is born prematurely, but only if the breathing is supported. This can be done by using supplemental oxygen while the baby lives in an incubator until they can breathe unassisted. In the term (not premature) baby the lungs are ready to use at 38 weeks, and they do continue to develop for a further eighteen months after birth, not reaching full maturity for another twenty-odd years.

While in the womb during the final trimester, the baby's diaphragm rhythmically contracts in a movement very much akin to breathing, despite the lungs being filled with amniotic fluid (the fluid surrounding the baby in the womb) and not air. This breathing occurs despite the fact that no gas exchange takes place. These breathing movements are only made between 18 and 60 per cent of the day.[4] The movements help develop the respiratory muscles and are essential for lung development. The frequency of the 'breaths' varies with age, decreasing as gestation progresses; they cease just before delivery. The breathing manoeuvres also change with the activity of the mother and the baby: for instance, they increase when the baby dreams (or is in REM sleep) and are more likely to occur during late evening and least likely at dawn.[5] Foetal hiccups are more pronounced than breathing and most mothers can feel these when pregnant. The difference between the sharp movements attributed to hiccups and the smooth undulations of breathing were first described medically in humans in 1888, but were not recorded in humans until 1971 by scientists using ultrasound.[6] When leaving the womb (and sometimes even during delivery), a baby will start breathing within a dozen or so seconds. How this transition between an aqueous and aerial medium occurs has baffled the greatest minds since ancient times. The crux of the issue was how the foetus survived for several months in the womb without breathing air and then switched instantly to being dependent on breathing air at birth.[7]

After birth, the umbilical cord connecting the mother to the child would not have gone unnoticed by our early ancestors, and nor would its association with the initiation of breathing once the cord was cut. To the ancient Greeks this provided a conduit through which pneuma could pass between the mother and baby. William Harvey (1578–1657) was the first to theorize in print upon this conundrum. His speculations are presented in his book *De generatione animalium*, published in 1651. Harvey wondered why a baby, once born, cannot survive without breathing after spending seven months in the womb without a single breath. This hinted to Harvey that the purpose of breathing air was not to regulate body temperature (as was the current theory in vogue at the time), but rather to foster combustion within the body, creating heat rather than dissipating it.

A later study on birth by the Scottish physician Robert Whytt, published as *On the Vital and Other Involuntary Motions of Animals* (1751), infers that the first breath resulted from a sensation or appetite in the baby akin to hunger or thirst, a sensation he described as the 'sentinel principal with which the body is endowed'. At birth the baby reacting to this sensation expands its chest and begins to breathe.[8] Many other theories existed: some suggested that it was the 'struggles' of birth that stimulated breathing, or the change in temperature upon leaving the womb. Another theory was that the beating heart created a vacuum around itself, causing the lungs to expand and start breathing. Albrecht von Haller (1708–1777), a Swiss physician, and Erasmus Darwin (1731–1802), English physician and grandfather to Charles, both independently thought that a baby's first breath was to do with the act of swallowing, with the baby wanting to feed upon birth. John Bostock (1773–1846), a physician from Liverpool, considered that it was due to the natural expansion of the baby after being compressed in the uterus. It wasn't until the twentieth century that the true reason was found.

Lung growth while in the womb is important. Recent evidence has shown that being born early with immature lungs can affect childhood in many ways. The lungs of those born prematurely (before 37 weeks of pregnancy) can develop less quickly in childhood than the lungs of children born at term (after 37 weeks). This can result in these children exhibiting reduced physical and cognitive abilities.[9] The consequences of early birth even track into adulthood. How early birth alters lung growth is still the subject of much research.[10]

Our lungs continue growing throughout our childhood and early adulthood, and reach their zenith by the time we enter our early twenties. After this, lung function is on a steady downward trend.

The ability to start breathing spontaneously upon birth, and its maintenance, has been used by many to advance arguments regarding the mechanisms of generation or evolution, as it cannot be a learnt function. Sometimes the argument is for acquired inheritance, as suggested by the French naturalist Jean-Baptiste Lamarck (1744–1829); sometimes it is for environmentally acquired inheritance, as suggested by the Russian biologist Trofim Lysenko

(1898–1976). Charles Darwin argued that innate functions such as breathing were preprogrammed, but that associated functions such as the ability to speak and sing were acquired.

OUR FIRST STEPS into the living world involve the rapid transition from a fluid-filled realm to a more nebulous and gaseous one. We gasp and begin breathing. Henceforth we are solely responsible, consciously or subconsciously, for ensuring that we supply ourselves with enough oxygen to live. This transition at birth to spontaneous and rhythmic breathing has fascinated humankind for millennia and was at first ascribed a spiritual explanation; it was supposed to provide evidence of the transfer of a vital life force from one generation to the next, from mother to child. While the beliefs regarding the function and purpose of breathing were similar across the ancient world, it took many centuries before breathing's true function was brought to light.

TWO

EARLY BELIEFS

O ur Neolithic ancestors would have been well aware of the act of breathing, so we should expect to find many cultural artefacts associated with breathing from this epoch. The opposite is true: archaeologists have found little. Most of the cave art from this period depicts animals and hunting scenes, from which nothing pertinent about breathing can be inferred. The nearest related artefacts are primitive wind instruments, flutes carved from bones, with the oldest being around 40,000 years old. Older archaeological evidence from the bones left behind have shown that our early human ancestors suffered from respiratory disease. In Turkey a fossilized *Homo erectus* skull dating from *c.* 510,000–490,000 years ago bears a lesion on its inner surface resulting from a tuberculosis infection.[1] Our history of breathing begins with the rise of the earliest civilizations, when knowledge was circulated via written texts, and when people first tried to make sense of the world through science, philosophy and religion.

Early Civilizations

Early civilizations did not understand breathing as we do today. It was viewed as an animating force possessing a spiritual vitality, with the back and forth of breathing providing the continuum of life.

The recorded human knowledge of breathing begins with the ancient Egyptians. The earliest medical papyri, from 2750 BC, reveal little about the biology of breathing, let alone any clear anatomical knowledge relating to the respiratory system. This is not surprising, as early Egyptian anatomical knowledge was associated more with the dead than the living, and concerned with the processes of mummification and embalming. In preparing bodies for burial the heart was considered the most important organ, and was often removed and placed in its own jar, which was stowed separately in the burial chamber. The lungs, which surround the heart, were placed in one of four canopic jars and given no further prominence. The Edwin Smith papyrus, a medical text from 1501 BC, mentions some canals in the chest which could be the bronchial tubes, while another medical text, the Ebers papyrus (1550 BC), mentions 'four vessels to the lungs and spleen.' Whether these are bronchial tubes or arteries is not clear.[2]

A few tomb glyphs thought to represent the lungs have been found since. The most convincing comes from the tomb of a nobleman, Pahery, in El-Kab and is from the Eighteenth Dynasty, dating to around the fifteenth century BC. The glyph is detailed enough to show the windpipe (trachea) with two bronchial tubes on either side lying atop the two lobes of the lung. While not anatomically correct, it is the earliest known image of the lung.[3]

Apart from the Egyptians, the early civilizations around Europe, Arabia, northern Africa and Asia considered that breathing fulfilled an important spiritual role. The Hellenistic philosophers and thinkers were the first to attempt a more factual explanation, which with modern hindsight looks no different to that expounded by their contemporary religious thinkers, be they Christian, Muslim or Hindu.

The ancients considered that the act of breathing, body heat and the air were all part of life's vital force. To the Greeks, breathing was elemental and not an integrated function. The atmosphere (air) and space occupied by the world was called the aether (modern spelling: ether). This aether was an immutable inert substance surrounding everything, different to the atmospheric air we know today. The moving air was felt as a blowing wind and breeze, and termed 'pneuma' (from the ancient Greek

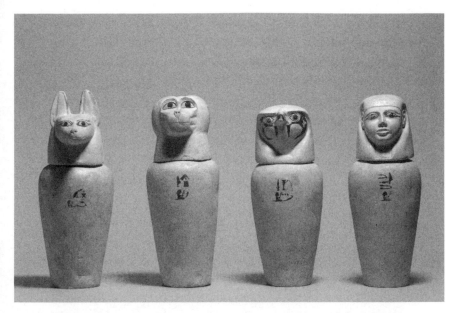

Egyptian canopic jars contained internal organs removed from the body during mummification. The lungs were placed in the jar depicting Hapi (second from the right), the baboon-headed son of Horus. This painted limestone example dates back to *c.* 900–800 BC (Third Intermediate Period).

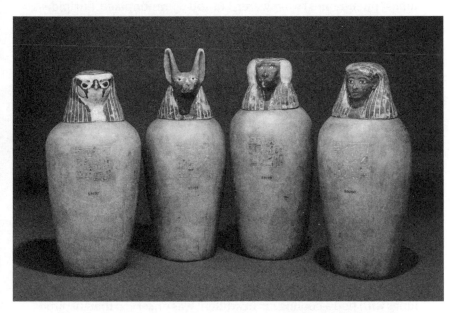

First Book of Breathing of Ousirour, *c.* 150–100 BC (Ptolemaic Period), papyrus. Throth is shown weighing the soul of Ousirour before Isis and Osiris (note the four canopic jars).

verb *pneo*).[4] Today we still use the derivations of this word to mean anything pertaining to the air, breathing or the lungs, for example in words such as 'pneumatic' and 'pneumonia'. To the early thinkers pneuma not only had physical meaning but was enmeshed with religious or spiritual dimensions. Thus aether and pneuma were separate things. Hippocrates (460–370 BC) accepted the idea that the body had essential components, of which pneuma (air) and water were two. Another humour was termed *calor* or fire but was better thought of as heat (body temperature); warmth signified life and cold denoted death. This heat was not thought of as fire but as a spirit similar in nature to the sun and stars. Thus heat and pneuma were part of the same thing, reflecting the vital force of life. Nowadays we know that body heat results from a myriad of complex chemical reactions occurring in cells, but back then it was thought that our breathing functioned to regulate this vital heat, cooling the inner heat generated by the beating heart, where the pneuma was thought to reside.[5]

To the public the difference between the air (pneuma) and lungs (pneumones) was clearer-cut and commonplace. Euripides (480–406 BC) in his tragic play *Orestes* stated that the pneuma comes from the lungs, while his contemporary Sophocles (c. 496–406 BC) in his tragedy *Trachiniae* or *The Maidens of Trachis* refers to the lungs as the most vital part of the body.

A more mechanistic view of breathing gradually evolved. This was first proposed by the Greek physician Empedocles (495–435 BC), whose ideas were influenced by his predecessors such as Pythagoras (570–495 BC). Empedocles' views on the role of respiration survive only as two dozen lines of poetry later passed on by the great philosopher and scientist Aristotle (384–322 BC). To Empedocles the air entered into the blood not only via the nose and mouth but through pores in the skin. Once in the blood, the fire it contained warmed the body. This warmth drove the first breath of the newborn infant; the breath's purpose was to fill the lungs with body-cooling air. In adults it was observed that inspired air was cool and expired air warm, and it was this constant cooling that maintained life, its interruption resulting in death. Empedocles further refined his notion by postulating that sleep is related to the heat of the blood; when blood is cooled sufficiently, it leads to sleep; where it is cooled too much, death results, and the body becomes cold and lifeless. Although vague, this does try to provide a rational explanation of how breathing changes with activity, as shallow, slow and regular breathing was associated with sleep, while increased activity engendered a feeling of overheating and resulted in faster and deeper breathing.

The early Greeks, like Empedocles, thought that life resulted from a combination of four forms of matter: earth, fire (calor) water and air (pneuma); and four qualities: dry, wet, hot and cold. These, when combined, gave the four vital humours of the body: blood, phlegm, yellow bile and black bile. Good health was represented by the balance of these humours, while ill health resulted from their imbalance.

Half a century later Aristotle proposed a more complicated explanation for breathing, as he thought that the humoral mechanistic view was far too simple. In his work *Peri anapoe* or *About Breath*, he postulated that pneuma was part of the animating spirit of life itself. In this case the brain housed one aspect of this spirit (consciousness or Thymos), while the pneuma provided the energy or fuel. Interrupting it led to death.

In the aftermath of the reign of Alexander the Great two Greek physicians, Herophilus (335–280 BC), an anatomist, and Erasistratus (310–250 BC), one of the first physiologists, who both lived in Alexandria, Egypt, were the first to try and link breathing to anatomy, developing a mechanistic view based on observation and an understanding of fundamental physics. The two observed that the chest wall expanded and contracted on its own independently of the lungs contained therein, an important observation at the time. Furthermore, they noted the association of specific muscles and nerves with the respiratory movements of breathing.

The Roman physician Galen (AD 129–210) was the next to make important contributions to our understanding of breathing. Importantly, he documented the discoveries and views of his predecessors, recording what they had said and written and saving this early knowledge for posterity. Even by Galen's time, many Greek manuscripts had been lost, and only fragments were left to comment upon, a few pages here, a passage there. As most texts were handwritten, few copies existed. Many texts were destroyed in fires, whether by accident or arson; the great library at Alexandria was burnt to the ground for the second time in AD 391 by Christians under order of the Roman emperor Theodosius, and many texts were lost during the Sack of Rome by King Alaric and the Visigoths in 410.

Galen's major contribution was made through his acute personal observational skills as a scientist, physician and record-keeper. Galen was born in Pergamon in Asia Minor into a wealthy merchant family. This independence allowed him to pursue a career in medicine. At that time Pergamon hosted one of the best medical schools in the ancient Western world, with a staff to match. Galen made the most of his four years at the Pergamon school until he left for a tour of Greece and northern Egypt. His clinical career began at the age of 27 on his return to Pergamon, where he became the physician to the gladiators.

Galen provided new insights into the mechanisms of breathing. As a physician, he witnessed the many injuries the soldiers received while fighting in the local wars or as gladiators. Galen observed how anatomy was related to function, recording the injuries the gladiators inflicted on one another. During some of these gladiatorial bouts, he observed that continued breathing was dependent on an intact brain and nervous system. He found that while a major frontal slash to the neck was often fatal, as the gladius (a short sword) would severe the windpipe or the carotid arteries, a slash to the rear of the neck less often resulted in death. He noted further that if a gladiator were slashed across the lower neck, he would rarely survive, and his breathing would instantly stop. A slash just a few centimetres higher was often survivable, even though the person might lose the use of his limbs. We now know that this is because the nerve centre that regulates our automatic breathing is based in the lower brain, called the medulla, which connects the spinal cord with the brain. A lower neck injury would slice through the nerves linking the brain stem with the lungs, removing the signals telling the respiratory muscles when to contract (breathe in) or relax (breathe out). Slicing the neck above the control centre allows the centre to continue sending signals to the respiratory muscles. Galen's observations were ahead of his time and it was not until the eighteenth century that the respiratory centre was located and discovered.

In the original Greek Bible, pneuma possessed a duality of function, the everyday and divine. Thus someone could possess simple human spirit (the everyday) or the divine spirit of God. This divine pneuma provided a person with oracular or prophetic abilities, one example being Balaam's donkey, which speaks with a human voice, the voice of God.[6] In the New Testament the Holy Spirit (pneuma) was instilled into the disciples of Jesus 'when he breathed on them, and saith unto them, Receive ye the Holy Ghost' (John 20:22). In later Christian theology and thinking this duality was lost and the soul and pneuma became one, with the pneuma becoming equivalent to the Holy Spirit. Pneumatology and spirituality are still important avenues of research and debate within the modern Christian Church.

While the Western world went on to develop a mechanistic explanation of breathing, the rest of the world, and in particular Asia, followed the more ethereal and spiritual beliefs that remain today and are manifested in the tradition of meditation. The Chinese also held the vitalist view, but saw breathing as an energy flow that could be controlled by exercise or meditation. This belief still influences many relaxation therapies practised in the West today. In other parts of Asia, particularly on the Indian subcontinent, these beliefs were reflected in the practice of Buddhist meditation.

In India medical knowledge progressed through the Ayurveda system and was recorded in compendia known as the Samhitas, written in Sanskrit around BC 400.[7] In these works, pneuma is known as prana, and according to the Sushruta Samhitas, 'Prana is neither vital air, nor air itself but the very energy that activates the elements abiding in the body.'[8] Prana is therefore intimately linked with breathing, and although it resides in the lungs and heart, it is exchanged during breathing. These Indian concepts, although subtly different to the Greek views, do reflect the notion that breathing has a spiritual rather than physiological function.

The medieval Persian physician Ibn Sina (981–1037), also known as Avicenna, contributed hugely to medicine through his book the *Canon of Medicine* (*Al-Qanun fi al-Tibb*). Published in 1025, it remained a leading source of knowledge for the next six hundred years.[9] The third volume of the *Canon* is titled 'Lungs and Chest', and while its five chapters describe in great detail the anatomy of the lungs, including the larynx (voice box) and chest wall, he did not link form with function. Without knowing the microscopic structure of the lungs or being aware of oxygen, he expounded the view that respiration was involved in cooling the blood. He was the first to comment on how breathing was related to health, and that disordered breathing was common in diseases such as asthma. He distinguished between breathing that was deep, shallow, fast, slow, warm and cold, for example, based on his observations. Many of his findings are still relevant today, but some are misguided, such as the belief that excessive sleeping and alcohol intake cause asthma. The *Canon* is important as it is one of the first texts to suggest that blood circulates through the lungs after expulsion from the right side of the heart before returning to the heart's left side. This pre-dates William Harvey's work by many centuries. The works of Ibn Sina, published in Arabic, were not translated and remained unknown in Europe, and were only rediscovered in the 1920s when an Egyptian physician, Muhyo Al-Deen el Tatawi, came across a manuscript copy of the *Canon* in the Prussian State Library in Berlin, Germany. Luckily, its importance was realized and it was subsequently translated into English, French and German.[10]

While the Occidental Roman Empire declined in Constantinople until its final collapse in 1453, Graeco-Roman medical knowledge was preserved in Persian medical schools, which were originally founded by the Assyrians in Mesopotamia. The school at Gondishapur founded in 555 ensured that the Graeco-Roman texts were translated into Syriac. With the fall of the Sasanian Empire of Persia in the seventh century, the coming of the Muslims led to the knowledge being disseminated across the Arab world, where medical schools were modelled on the Persian ones. At this time the Arab empire reached into Spain and Portugal, and it was here that many medical texts were copied into Greek by Benedictine monks. Here they remained until the foundation of the first European medical schools. One of the earliest appeared in tenth-century Italy at Salerno. The translated Greek texts were restored from the monasteries and translated into Latin, beginning a renaissance in the study of anatomy, first with animal and then human dissection.[11]

Medieval to Renaissance

The study of breathing in Europe was piecemeal. In the twelfth century one Master Nicolaus, a Polish monk, stated that the lungs were hollow in order to retain air 'for cooling the heart and renewing the vital spirits'. Three hundred years later Michael Servetus (1511–1553), a Spanish theologian and physician, independently rediscovered the findings made by Ibn Sina. Servetus's religious views were considered heretical at the time by both Protestants and Catholics. In 1553, while living incognito in Strasbourg, Servetus published the book *Christianismi restitutio* or *Christianity Restored*, detailing these heretical views. It was in this book that Servetus also included his theories and description of the pulmonary circulation and its function. Unwisely, he sent a copy of his book to the theologian and reformer John Calvin in Geneva, who rejected the work outright and threatened him with death if he ever came to visit him in Switzerland. During that summer, leaving Strasbourg and with the intention of moving to Italy, Servetus's route took him via Geneva. He took the opportunity to visit the city but was quickly recognized and imprisoned. At first the Genevans did not know what to do with Servetus and it was some weeks before they decided he should be executed. In October he was burned at the stake with a copy of his book strapped to his leg.[12] Calvin ordered that all copies of the book be destroyed, intending that Servetus's views should die with him. Fortunately, a few copies survived in obscurity. This isn't the end of the tale, as in the 1950s one of the surviving books was re-examined by an American historian. Servetus's pulmonary writings were rediscovered and brought back to the attention of modern scholars.

The great Italian anatomist, scientist and artist Leonardo da Vinci (1452–1519) produced detailed images of the lungs and speculated on their function and the role of breathing: 'From the heart, sooty vapours are carried back to the lung by way of the pulmonary artery to be exhaled to the outer air.'[13]

During this era, a new breed of exploratory anatomists appeared, such as the Italian Jacopo Berengario da Carpi (1466–1530) and the Frenchman Charles Estienne (c. 1505–1564), all of whom began to provide a detailed anatomy of the body and to systematically name the anatomical structures they so carefully dissected. And it was not until the sixteenth century, with the great Italian anatomists Sylvius Fallopius Hieronymus Fabricius (1533–1619) and Andreas Vesalius (1514–1564) of the University of Padua, that the view of pneuma was challenged. Returning to dissection and close examination of the heart and lungs provided them with the hint that Galen's view of circulation was incorrect; and that blood circulated from the right side of the heart through the lungs and back to the left side, and thence on through the body; and that air was found only outside the body.[14] These theories were finally proved correct by the seventeenth-century studies of the English physician William Harvey. Harvey, who worked closely with living animals, established beyond doubt that blood passed from the arteries into veins, through which it returned to the heart. These studies were a major breakthrough, in that the system under investigation was best observed in vivo (in live animals, using vivisection), when the physiological conditions could be manipulated, which allowed the anatomical features under investigation to be better understood. Harvey's discoveries can be said to be on a par with Isaac Newton's later, more renowned, elucidation of gravity.

Despite these great advances, Harvey did not provide any new insights into the purpose of breathing. He wrote: It must be either because the larger and more perfect animals are warmer, and when adult their heat greater – ignited, as I might say, and requiring to be damped or mitigated; therefore it may be that the blood is sent through the lungs, that it may be tempered by the air that is inspired, and prevented from boiling up, and so becoming extinguished, or something else of the sort.' Later in life, Harvey was embarrassed by not knowing why blood circulated, stating that 'I own I am of the Opinion that our first duty is to inquire whether the thing be or not, before asking wherefore it is.' In 1616 he noted: '1. Do the Lungs have a special function at all? 2. If they have a special function, is it of the nature of alteration or heating or cooling? 3. What is the basis of this alteration and what does it do with each of blood, air and spirit?'[15]

Resolving the conundrum of the purpose of breathing was hindered by the lack of detailed knowledge of lung structure. The Greeks knew that the lungs were spongelike and resembled the granular or lobular structure of the liver and pancreas. They also knew that, just as in the liver, a great many blood vessels, some quite large, traverse the lungs. Thus it was reasoned that the lungs and liver formed from the blood, a light and foamy fraction in the lungs and a heavy and thick fraction in the liver. This view was not only expounded by Andreas Vesalius but by Harvey, who claimed that the only difference between the lungs and liver is one of density. Close visual inspection of the lungs could provide only limited detail of their anatomic structure, even when magnifying glasses were used, so it wasn't until the microscope was invented that the ultra-fine detail of lung tissue could be examined and the function of breathing interrogated further.

The first person to use a microscope to examine the lungs and report his findings was the Italian anatomist Marcello Malpighi. Using his primitive microscope to examine frog lungs, he was able to observe and illustrate the lungs' finest structures, the alveoli or air sacs. He reported his findings to his friend Counsellor Alfonso Borelli in two long open letters, which were later published as

De pulmonibus in Florence in 1661. In the first, he stated, 'I have discovered that the whole mass of lung to which [we] are attached the excurrent vessels, is an aggregate of very fine membranes which, stretched and folded, form an almost infinite number of orbicular bladders.' He thought these bladders resembled the hexagonal honeycomb structure found in beehives. We now know that these bladders or air sacs represent the functional unit of the lung where gas exchange between the air and blood takes place. Malpighi further saw that the air-filled windpipe or trachea branched first into two, and then four, and then eight and so on into ever finer tubes until they merged with his 'orbicular bladders', thus linking the outside air with these fine structures.

His second epistle continues to describe how blood flows through the lungs and subsequently details for the first time the capillaries, the exceedingly small vessels that link the arteries to the veins, finally shedding light on how blood circulated around the body without having to go through some mysterious transformation in the organs and muscles. This discovery provided a new explanation for the purpose of breathing, as Malpighi thought that the expansion and contraction of the lungs was intended to mix, knead and squeeze the blood through the soft lungs and aid its return to the heart.

The question of why the lungs inflate and deflate was investigated by the English scientist Robert Hooke (1635–1703), a practical man who excelled at experimentation. He was a polymath who contributed to many disciplines during his life, applying his knowledge and expertise to each new venture he chose. He is famous for his illustrations of microscopic views of living material, published in his book *Micrographia* (1665). While at the University of Oxford working with the English scientist Robert Boyle, who was investigating the physics of air, Hooke performed his own studies on breathing in animals. In 1667, aged 32, he showed, using a complex system of bellows to ventilate the static lungs, that fresh air was needed to keep an animal alive, and that it was not just the movement of the chest walls that was required. At the same time, he was working with the physician Richard Lower, who noticed that blood changed colour as it passed through the ventilated lungs, changing from a burgundy red to a bright scarlet, and that this change in colour was independent of whether the animal was alive or not. These studies showed that air contained something which Lower termed 'nitrous spirit'. The observation that breathing provided a vital agent which was not supplied by the pumping heart was the first evidence that the lungs and breathing performed their own intrinsic function. The lungs were not there to cool the blood or help pump it around the body.

By the seventeenth century air was no longer considered an ethereal force, like wind, but a physical entity with physical properties such as density and pressure, although its exact chemical composition still remained a mystery. Even a clear definition of air was lacking. Boyle, in his treatise *The General History of the Air* (1692), states: 'By the Air, I commonly understand that thin diaphanous, compressible and dilatable Body in which we breathe and wherein we live.' Here the term 'body' means the atmosphere.

Today we know that the atmosphere is made up of numerous gases, mainly nitrogen, oxygen, argon and carbon dioxide. These gases (with the exception of argon), when combined with other elements such as hydrogen and carbon, make up 93 per cent of its mass. As elements, oxygen is represented by the chemical symbol O, hydrogen by the letter H, and carbon by the letter C. Gaseous oxygen in its natural form consists of two atoms bound together (it is one of seven diatomic gas molecules), called dioxygen and denoted O_2.

Once dissolved in the blood, oxygen is transported to cells, where it is immediately used to generate energy, powering the body's metabolism. Extraordinarily little oxygen is stored in the body, hence our need to breathe constantly. Oxygen is used to burn organic compounds such as fat and sugar, and generates energy-containing compounds such as ATP (adenosine triphosphate). A by-product of these chemical reactions is the generation of heat, which warms our blood and bodies. The energy content gained through reacting with oxygen is measured in calories, the units we associate with our food. Once the oxygen has passed through a series of complex chemical reactions, the two oxygen atoms end up combined with carbon (derived from our food), forming the waste gas carbon dioxide (CO_2), or a single atom may combine with hydrogen to form a water molecule (H_2O). Unlike diatomic oxygen, CO_2 dissolves readily in water, which is fortunate, as this allows the waste CO_2 to pass easily into the blood. Within a few minutes all the blood will eventually pass through the lungs via the capillaries in the alveoli, where it comes into close contact with the alveolar air. This air, although damp and warm, contains hardly any CO_2, so the CO_2 fluxes quickly across from the CO_2-laden blood into the alveoli and is expired back into the outside air.

All three compounds, oxygen, carbon dioxide and water, are toxic in too large a quantity. Oxygen is too energetic on its own, even more so as a solo atom, so high cellular concentrations will damage the cells. For example, if premature babies are given too much oxygen, it can cause blindness and damage the lungs. The solubility of carbon dioxide and its propensity to dissolve into water means that it can form an electrically charged polyatomic compound, hydrogen carbonate, often called bicarbonate (HCO_3). This is how most of the metabolized carbon dioxide is carried in the blood. The problem is that the hydrogen in this compound can free itself from it, and not in its natural diatomic form, H_2, but as a single positively charged atom, H^+. This form of hydrogen is very reactive and in high concentrations makes solutions more acidic. Unfortunately, our tissues do not thrive in highly acidic environments, hence its toxicity. Thus the processes of breathing, pulmonary ventilation and cellular respiration work together to supply oxygen to the cells and expel the used oxygen, in combination with carbon and hydrogen. Removing the food-derived carbon via CO_2 is one of the main ways we lose weight, as carbon is not readily removed in the urine.

It was a contemporary of Boyle, the Cornishman and physiologist John Mayow (1641–1679), who discovered that air was not a single compound and consisted of two portions: one that supported combustion, which he called nitro-aereus (oxygen), and one that did not. By placing mice or burning candles in sealed jars, he demonstrated that nitro-aereus (oxygen) was also consumed during breathing (and by flames), leading him to postulate that particles of nitro-aereus were transported in the blood where they underwent combustion in the body to produce heat. He published his work in the *Tractatus quinque medico-physici* (1674), which consists of five treatises in Latin, one of which is on respiration. Unfortunately he died young, in his late thirties, and his work was soon forgotten.

Post-Renaissance to the Eighteenth Century

Mayow's treatise lay dormant on library shelves for some 120 years before it was rediscovered in 1790 by the physician and science writer Dr Thomas Beddoes (1760–1808). With Mayow's work unknown at the time, the phlogiston theory had provided the most convincing explanation of air's dual nature. This theory had been proposed principally by the German chemist Johann Joachim Becher in 1667. The theory was based on Empedocles' idea of the four elements of earth, water, wind and fire. The idea was that the air contained a flammable substance known as phlogiston (from the ancient Greek for 'burning up'), which when burned turned to dephlogisticated air, which was non-flammable. Animals and plants were thought to absorb the phlogiston and create dephlogisticated air; this explained why wood would burn when later placed in a fire, as it was thought to contain phlogiston.

The idea of the chemical elements was becoming popular, so many scientists set out to try and discover the identity of phlogiston. This was achieved by three European scientists. In 1772 Carl Wilhelm Scheele (1742–1786), a Swedish chemist, discovered oxygen, which he called fire-air, publishing his findings in 1777 in a pamphlet, *Abhandlung von der Luft und dem Feuer* (Treatise on Air and Fire). In the meantime, a Scottish chemist, polymath, minister and teacher, Joseph Priestley (1733–1804), independently discovered oxygen, which he called 'dephlogisticated air' (and not phlogiston). He was slow to report his discovery in *Experiments*

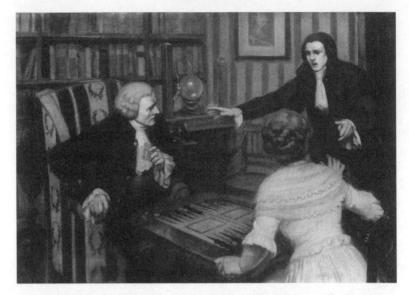

Ernest Board, *Joseph Priestley, the Discoverer of Oxygen*, 1912, oil on canvas. Priestley is depicted in his Birmingham home at the moment he receives the news that it is about to be attacked by an anti-radical mob.

and Observations on Different Kinds of Air, released in six volumes (1774–86). In 1774 Priestley visited the prominent French chemist Antoine Lavoisier (1743–1794) in Paris, where he demonstrated his recent discovery of oxygen. Lavoisier was impressed by Priestley's work and conducted his own experiments, giving him the insight to make the intellectual jump of defining oxygen as a new chemical element, of which there were around seventeen others known at the time. Lavoisier then refuted the phlogiston theory in his book *Réflexions sur le phlogistique* (1783). He did not fully understand oxygen and mistakenly thought that it was generated from acids, hence his name for the element, *oxygène* (from the Greek term for 'sharp-producing'). Lavoisier and his wife, Marie-Anne, who was also a chemist, went on to conduct many more studies on oxygen and breathing. As well as a chemist, Lavoisier was a noble-man with radical ideas living in revolutionary times. The French Revolution proved his undoing: as an unpopular aristocrat and tax administrator he was charged with tax fraud and sentenced to death. He was executed by guillotine in 1794 at the age of fifty. The mathematician Joseph-Louis LaGrange (1736–1813), a contemporary, lamented the beheading, stating, 'It took them only an instant to cut off that head, but France may not produce another like it in a century.'[16]

In the meantime, Joseph Black (1728–1799), a Scottish chemist, (re)discovered carbon dioxide, calling it 'fixed air (CO_2)', although it had been described a hundred years earlier by the Dutchman Jan Baptiste van Helmont. In 1754 Black found, through a series of experiments involving mixing and heating chalk, magnesium salts and acid, that a gas was released, which he identified by measuring how much weight the original mixture had lost. Joseph Priestley, who in the 1760s lived near a brewery in Leeds, noticed the large amount of 'fixed air' generated during fermentation. It was not until 1799 that oxygen and carbon dioxide were confirmed to be present in the blood by Sir Humphry Davy (1778–1829), who at the age of 21 was working in Penzance, Cornwall, as a physician's assistant. Davy collected the gases that were emitted from heated blood. He also made other discoveries: he gave the elemental gas chlorine its name, after its colour, as derived from the Greek *chloros*, meaning green-yellow. It had originally been discovered by Scheele in 1774, who had called it 'dephlogisticated marine air', thinking it was a compound of oxygen. (The impact of chlorine on our cultural history and the history of breathing must wait until the twentieth century.)

With these advances in chemistry and physics, a new mechanistic view of breathing and medicine emerged across Europe. In the UK one new and influential system of medicine was advocated by two influential Scottish physicians, first William Cullen (1710–1790) and then his younger protégé John Brown (1735–1788). Cullen believed that the nervous system was the focal point of disease in the body, and he began to classify diseases as being caused by either too much stimulation or too much sedation of the nervous system. Brown extended and simplified this idea further, believing that all disease was due to an unbalanced physiology, and published his ideas in *Elementa medicinae* in 1780. This was a step too far for Cullen, and he and Brown acrimoniously parted company. Cullen's and Brown's views about the pharmacological properties of opium were opposite: Cullen and his followers, the Cullenians, argued that it was a sedative, while the Brunonians perceived it as a stimulant. On either view, diseases such as pneumonia, whooping cough and asthma were considered weaknesses of the body, so treatment could be obtained by stimulation or excitement, and were treated with powerful emetics such as syrup of ipecac, which when ingested resulted in violent vomiting. While the Cullenian viewpoint floundered, Brunonian medicine, as it was called, became popular in Europe and North America, appealing to younger physicians who had ideas of revolution and reformation uppermost in their minds. Seeking his fortune, Brown left Scotland in 1786 for London, where he died two years later of a stroke.

The English physician Thomas Beddoes believed in Brunonian medicine and experimented with the recently discovered gases oxygen, hydrogen and carbon dioxide. He believed that excitation was achieved by breathing oxygen and sedation by using other gases, such as carbon dioxide. This oxygen-centred view reflected the recent discoveries of Priestley and Lavoisier, whom he had met in his travels and as a student. Beddoes attributed scurvy and obesity to a deficiency of oxygen and tuberculosis and bronchitis to an excess of oxygen. Thus fresh air could be used to treat scurvy, and a lowered oxygen intake would treat respiratory disease. The lowering of oxygen was achieved by adding 'harmless gases' such as azotic (nitrogen), hydrogene (hydrogen) and carbonic air (carbon dioxide). Beddoes believed that adding hydrogen was the best way of downgrading the effect of oxygen. He pursued his research alongside Humphry Davy at the newly founded Pneumatic Institute in Bristol, sometime later called the Medical Institution for the Sick and Drooping Poor. At the Pneumatic Institute it was common to try the gas mixtures on employees and non-fee-paying patients. Davy promoted the gas nitrous oxide for its anaesthetic properties, but also for its euphoric properties. When inhaled with air it made people feel light-headed, giving rise to the nickname 'laughing gas', and by the 1800s 'laughing gas parties' were popular among the wealthy.

The audience at a
lecture enjoying the
effects of 'laughing
gas' (nitrous oxide).
Illustration by
George Cruikshank
for John Scoffern,
*Chemistry No
Mystery; or,
A Lecturer's
Bequest* (1834).

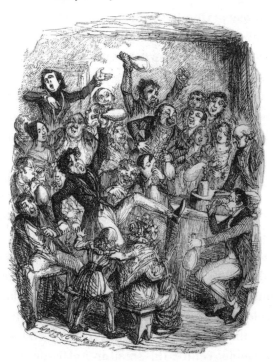

Beddoes was joined in this quest by the Scottish mechanical engineer and inventor James Watt, now considered one of the greatest contributors to the Industrial Revolution. Watt had lost his daughter Janet (Jessy) to tuberculosis in 1794 and his son Gregory later died of the infection in 1804. Driven by grief from his daughter's death, he sought a way to prevent the disease Watt also held Brunonian views and believed in Beddoes's 'chemistry of airs' as a promising way forward. He believed that adding hydrogen to the inspired air would reduce the symptoms of tuberculosis. To this end he experimented with methods of making hydrogen and then building respirators by which the gas could be safely added to the inspired air. Their motto was 'Inhale it and see.' Beddoes quickly concluded that adding other gases was not a good idea and suggested that only oxygen should be used, eventually losing his enthusiasm for the Brunonian doctrine, while Watt continued with these views and continued to experiment with other gases such as carbon dioxide. The two finally produced a book together, *Considerations on the Medicinal Use of Factitious Airs, and the*

Manner of Obtaining them in Large Quantities. It was published in two parts, the first by Beddoes and the second by Watt, in 1794. Watt died at the age of 83, while Beddoes, who was obese, died at 48 from a cardiac arrest.

Alongside these investigations, great advances were being made in neurology, leading to new observations regarding the rhythms and patterns of breathing. Galen had noted that when the nerves of animals were cut it altered their breathing, with the cutting of different nerves inducing different effects. The nerves in question are the phrenic (which causes the diaphragm to contract) and intercostal nerves; cutting the latter results in pain and the former in paralysis. Galen built on the observations of Herophilus and Erasistratus, who had noted that the contraction and relaxation of the diaphragm (the principle respiratory muscle) was important in breathing, as was the rising and falling of the ribcage. Galen's observations of gladiator injuries provided the first clue that the brain stem controls breathing and is the location of the 'breathing centre'. This small area of tissue in the medulla controls the rhythm and pattern of breathing. It is different from the control of the heartbeat rhythm, which is also regulated from a small area of tissue in the brain stem. Unlike the lungs, the heart contains its own independent pacemaker, so can beat independently of the brain and will beat spontaneously even when removed from the chest. Breathing stops as soon as the brain stem loses nervous contact with the respiratory muscles, such as the diaphragm. Today we know a lot more about the respiratory centre, its position in the medulla and how it provides our urge to breathe and the sensation of breathlessness. We know that injury to the spinal cord between region C1 and C4 (vertebrae) will impede breathing, and if the damage is serious breathing will need to be supported. Injuries lower down the spine, however, at C5 and C6, only weaken breathing, allowing the person to continue to breathe unassisted.

Both Leonardo da Vinci and Vesalius performed detailed dissections of the thorax. Leonardo's illustrations of lung dissections from 1508 and 1509 show the diaphragm, which he called the *djaflamma*, while his illustration of the dissected spinal cord, which he termed the 'tree of nerves', shows the spinal nerves and the intercostal nerves but not the phrenic nerve. This was not shown until Vesalius's 'nerve-man' illustration of 1543, which shows both the phrenic and intercostal nerves.

The Scottish physician and neurologist Robert Whytt was interested in the nervous system and the phenomenon of reflex reactions.[17] The common view still held that nervous action was mediated via pneuma (the vital animal spirit) and that some sentient force operating throughout the body was responsible for the operation of the body. In this context the act of breathing was considered a reflex reaction. It was an automatic process, for which there was a 'hunger or appetite'. This 'hunger' could be temporarily controlled by holding the breath, but it could not be overcome. It was already known through Galen that breathing was controlled by the medulla, but now it was understood that some of this function was located away from the brain in the lungs, and that the brain received functional feedback from the lungs.[18]

During this period, particularly in France, the aim was to locate the home of this urge to breathe, both in the spiritual and the anatomical sense. Breathing, along with a beating heart, was considered a vital sign of life, and the absence of the two defined death. The English physician and influential anatomist Thomas Willis (1621–1675) had wrongly located the respiratory centre in the cerebellum, a small body of nerves at the base and rear of the brain, overlooking Galen's work. Thus it was through a triangulation of studies by three French physicians and physiologist that the respiratory centre's true location was rediscovered: Anne-Charles Lorry (1726–1783), followed by Julien Jean César Le Gallois (1770–1814) and then Marie-Jean-Pierre Flourens (1794–1867). Lorry, who led by systematically removing slices of the brain until no brain was left, proved that the 'seat of life' was not in the 'Bony skull' – that is, the brain – but in the spinal cord. He found that his experimental animals (cats) breathed without a brain but that when he cut the spinal cord the animal ceased breathing. His work moved the respiratory centre from the cerebellum to an area between the first and forth vertebrae of the spinal cord.[19]

Next, Le Gallois, using headless freshly guillotined rabbits, was able to show that the respiratory centre was located even more precisely near the origin of the eighth pair of nerves. This work was followed by Flourens, who used crude ablation experiments wherein he would destroy parts of the brain, and showed that destroying the medulla oblongata in rabbits caused death. This showed how essential this tissue was for breathing and blood circulation.[20] Flourens called this area the *noeud vital* (vital node). While he had located the tissue that controlled breathing, it did not answer the philosophical question about the force of life.

Today our understanding of the control of breathing continues to grow. Important patches of nervous tissue associated with this respiratory centre are still being discovered and described. One such area is the Bötzinger and pre-Bötzinger complexes, described by Jack L. Feldman and his colleagues from the University of California, Los Angeles, and the University of Göttingen, Germany, in 1991. The public naming of these complexes was made impulsively by Feldman, who wanted to pre-empt a rival fellow scientist from naming them after himself. While announcing his discovery of the complex at a conference in Germany, he spotted on a table close by a wine bottle from the Bötzinger winery (a popular brand of wine from Baden), so he decided then and there to name the new cells the Bötzinger complex, fixing the name for evermore.

While the anatomical hunt for the respiratory centre was underway, parallel studies were being conducted on how nervous activity altered breathing patterns and rhythm. One peculiar abnormal form of breathing is Cheyne-Stokes breathing. This breathing pattern is seen only when the supply of oxygen and exhalation of carbon dioxide is disturbed, and can be pathological (for example, from heart failure) or due to the environment (for example, from sleeping at high altitude). It was first described in 1809 by John Cheyne (1777–1836), a Scottish physician and surgeon who was interested in croup (an inflammation of the trachea, causing a barking cough and hoarse voice), in his book *On the Pathology of the Membrane of the Larynx and Bronchia*, his co-author being Sir William Stokes (1804–1878), an Irish physician. The pair met in Ireland, where Cheyne had moved to Dublin to find his fame and fortune.[21] Cheyne-Stokes breathing is unusual, as it cycles first with a gradual increase in the volume of each breath until a crescendo is reached, and then the volume per breath gradually decreases (a decrescendo is reached). Breathing stops for a few seconds (apnoea) and starts all over again, repeating the cycle.

The name became more widely known after 1953 when Soviet Union state broadcasters, rather than reporting the impending death of Joseph Stalin, stated instead that he had fallen into Cheyne-Stokes breathing. At the time, few members of the public realized what this meant, but a young mathematician, Yuri Gastev, who was a long-term patient in hospital suffering from tuberculosis, overheard a doctor say that this meant it was the end for the unpopular leader. On hearing this a celebration ensued on the ward. After leaving hospital, every year Yuri and his friends toasted Cheyne and Stokes. Later in his career, when Yuri was working on a book he had written on cybernetics, he added the reference 'J. Cheyne and W. Stokes: The Breath of Death Marks the Rebirth of Spirit-mind, March 1953'. Five thousand copies of the book were printed and distributed before the Soviet authorities spotted the joke and withdrew the publication. In reprisal, Yuri's editor lost his job. Yuri escaped being fired as he had already been fired earlier by the publishers.[22]

Another pair of scientists who contributed to the story of breathing were the German physicians Karl Ewald Konstantin Hering (1834–1918) and Josef Breuer (1842–1925). Their paper 'The Self-steering of Respiration via the Vagus Nerve' was published in 1868. Hering and Breuer discovered that when we breathe in and the lung inflates, the output of the phrenic nerve serving the lungs is inhibited, thus slowing inflation. This negative feedback prevents the lungs from being overinflated. This system is now named the Hering–Breuer reflex. The doctors are today remembered for what to them was, at the time, a peripheral discovery, as Hering was better known for his work on colour vison, while

Breuer was an associate of Sigmund Freud, with whom he jointly published a book that was influential in the development of psychoanalysis, *Studien über Hysterie* (Studies on Hysteria, 1895). However, in respiratory matters Hering was the senior partner, although he was only eight years older, so his name precedes Breuer's. Hering had a son, Heinrich Ewald (1866–1948), who also became a physician and later studied the vagal control of the heart. Although he was only two years old when his father's paper was published, he has been wrongly accredited by several authors with the discovery of his father's reflex, even as recently as 2014.

In the history of understanding breathing, another important question regards what causes breathing to stop. The English physician Edmund Goodwyn (1756–1829) was only indirectly interested in the mechanisms of breathing; he was more interested in *not* breathing, or more precisely drowning, submersion and strangulation, as the very long title of his book of 1788 shows: *The Connexion of Life with Respiration; or, An Experimental Inquiry into the Effects of Submersion, Strangulation and Several Kinds of Noxious Airs, on Living Animals: with an Account of the Nature of Disease They Produce; Its Distinction from Death Itself; and the Most Effectual Means of Cure.*

He and his fellow scientists were investigating the cause of death from drowning; at the time asphyxiation – that is, lack of oxygen – would not have been considered a cause. Drowning was considered to result from nervous inactivity engendered by immersion in cold water. The reasoning behind this was expounded by the English surgeon Sir Anthony Carlisle (1768–1840) in his second Royal Society's Croonian Lecture on muscular motion in 1805. He observed that some animals hibernate when the temperature is cold, and postulated that those animals should be also resistant to drowning, through a peculiarity of their nervous system being suspended, along with respiration, when exposed to lower temperatures. He provided support to his ideas by describing his studies on submerged 'Hybernating hedge-hogs'. In these studies, one full-grown hedgehog in a state of hibernation survived thirty minutes submerged in a bowl of cold water, fully curled up, while another animal not in the state of hibernation only survived ten minutes in a bowl of warm water and died limp, 'relaxed and extended.'

These various strands of research, providing ever clearer insights into the biology of breathing, progressed as the details of the finer structure of the lungs were scaled up to provide an 'engineer's' view of breathing: the lungs being a pump that rely on

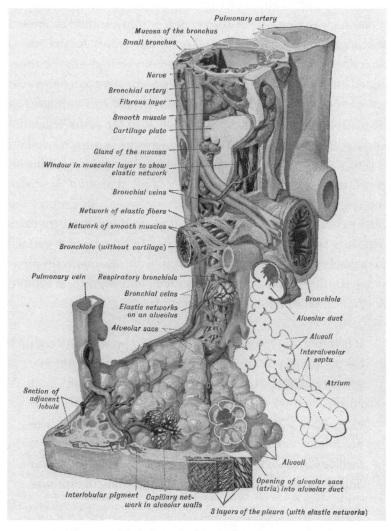

A pulmonary lobule from the lungs of a young man showing the close proximity of the airways, arteries and veins.
Plate from the *Textbook of Histology* (1943).

pressure and diffusion to work. The lungs are the largest organ in the body in terms of surface area, larger than the skin, for instance, which boasts an average surface area of 1.7 square metres all told in the average man. This task has not yet been achieved, but various indirect methods of measuring the surface area of the lungs have been found, some using biomathematical models and more recently X-ray CT scanners. Some of the earliest estimates were made by Gustav von Hüfner (1840–1908), professor of physiological chemistry in Tubingen, Germany. Hüfner estimated the lungs' total surface area to be 140 square metres. As Sir Charles Sherrington (1857–1952), a prominent physiologist of the time, stated, this is 'around 1,000 square feet, equivalent to a room with a floor space of 50 feet long and 20 feet wide.'[23] This estimate has been modified many times since, such as in the 1970s, when the surface area was likened to the area of a tennis court. Nowadays it is thought more to represent the area of a singles badminton court (dimensions 17 × 44 ft or 5.2 × 13.4 m) at around 70 square metres. Folded up, this surface encompasses only around 4–6 litres in volume, but serves to gives all 300 million alveoli intimate exposure to air and blood. It is not just the spectacular surface area that is impressive but the thinness of the alveolar walls separating the air from the blood. They are incredibly thin, at around 300 nanometres. In Sherrington's words,

> It is important to realise that the blood passing through the pulmonary artery (blood entering the lungs) suddenly spreads out into a layer which is not more than one blood corpuscle thick and is exposed to the air over this huge area, whence it is picked up again and collected into the pulmonary veins (and back to the heart). Such a means of facilitating rapid interchange of gases between the blood and a given volume of air we cannot possibly imitate artificially.[24]

These alveoli are connected together with around 2,400 km (1,500 mi.) of airways, and an even greater length of capillaries.

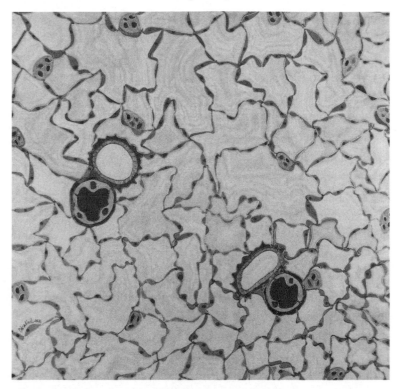

Odra Noel, *Deep Breath Respiratory Tissue*, n.d., paint on silk. The majority of the lungs are made up of very small alveoli forming a spongelike structure of air spaces.

Strength and elasticity are important as well. When inflating a balloon, you inhale deeply, filling all the air spaces in your lungs. Elasticity allows you to exhale forcibly into the balloon, creating positive pressure by contracting your respiratory muscles. Robust membranes are required, as it would be catastrophic if the lungs were torn apart. Thus the very thin alveolar wall has a four-ply structure.[25] This provides strength and lets gas exchange occur efficiently. The structure reduces the effects of gravity. We are unique among animals in that we stand upright, except when we sleep. In most mammals the lungs are level, but in humans the base and apex of the lungs are on the same horizontal plane. Gravity becomes important, as by its very nature lung tissue is exceptionally light, consisting mostly of air-filled tubes and spaces, but at the same time it is filled with around a litre of blood, the weight of which stresses the tissue, resulting in the base of the lungs receiving more ventilation than the apex.

It is one of nature's wonders that our resting breathing rate obeys a scaling law: the smaller the animal, the faster it breathes. Humans are medium-sized mammals, with adult bodies weighing on average between 50 and 100 kg (110 and 220 lb), and a resting breathing rate of around 14–20 breaths a minute. Compare this to the 2-gram Etruscan shrew (*Suncus etruscus*), which breathes at an incredibly fast rate of 600–700 breaths per minute,[26] while whales, such as the blue whale weighing 150,000 kg (330,700 lb), breathe through blowholes in the back of their throats only once a minute, or even once every two minutes, and can hold their breath easily for 30–90 minutes.[27]

Height, like body size, is related to breathing rate. In *Gulliver's Travels* (1726) by Jonathan Swift, Captain Lemuel Gulliver meets the Lilliputians, a race of tiny humans whom Gulliver estimates to be about the size of his index finger, around 14 centimetres tall (5½ in.). Being this small, their breathing rate should be 68 per minute, the same as a newborn baby.[28] Later, Gulliver meet the less well-known giant Brobdingnagians, who are estimated to be 20.5 metres (67 ft) high, giving them a breathing rate of five breaths per minute, about the same as a resting elephant. This change in breathing rate with size is seen as we grow up and mature: in newborn babies the rate is around 68 breaths per minute. Many first-time parents become concerned when they first notice this. By six months it is has reduced to a range of 25–40 breaths per minute, and continues to fall (at three, six and ten years old it is 20–30, 18–25 and 17–23 breaths per minute, respectively) until adulthood, when it reaches the adult range of 14–20 breaths per minute. Thereafter it stays stable until the efficiency of gas exchange declines and breathlessness increases the rate. Accompanying this fall in breathing rate with age is an increase in lung size, which follows growth in height: thus in a young male of around 1 metre (3 ft) in height the lungs are around 1.8 litres in volume, which by 1.5 metres (5 ft) increases to around 3.5 litres (with females having smaller volumes at equivalent heights).

By the nineteenth century, it was universally accepted that the purpose of breathing was to exchange oxygen for carbon dioxide, with the brain balancing this exchange through alteration of breathing rate and rhythm.

As increasingly careful measurements of breathing were made, it was noted that there was almost always an imbalance between the inspired and expired volume. It was still not clear what oxygen did once in the lungs, blood and tissues. Some scientists believed that oxygen was used in the digestive system, where food was 'combusted', while others believed oxygen acted on the lungs only and created a change in the blood, which then fuelled the production of heat. Others thought that the imbalance between the inspiration of oxygen and carbon dioxide could be accounted for by the lung converting some of the inspired oxygen into water, or even that nitrogen was actively respired.

The quest to solve this problem became fashionable among many young scientists, who were keen to clarify the many conflicting theories. To resolve these issues required careful measurement of the volumes and concentration of the inspired and expired air. The imbalance between the oxygen consumed and carbon dioxide produced became known as the respiratory quotient, and was around 0.8, meaning the expired volume was smaller than the inspired volume. The idea that food was burnt in the body stimulated the search for soot in the body. A Dr Pearson reported in 1813 that post-mortem lungs were often 'uniformly black' in people aged 65 and upwards and had a 'mottled or marbled appearance, from black and dark blue spots' in people aged around twenty.[29] Pearson analysed this 'mysterious' black carbonaceous substance and concluded that it was probably soot, and not some mysterious metabolite of oxygen consumption. Healthy lungs appear pink whatever the age. Pearson's false lead, rather than providing insight into the mysteries of oxygen consumption, show instead how polluted the air was at the time.

For much of the century breathing research would be dominated by Edinburgh and Paris. Major advances were made not just by physicians, but by chemists and physicists. The concept of 'vitalism' now being shunned, it was an optimistic age, when it was thought that chemical equations and physical laws alone could fully explain life. These new Victorians and French Republicans sought to explain the function of the lungs; physicists in terms of the recently discovered gas laws, with gas moving by diffusion, while chemists considered respiration to be a form of combustion producing heat. With the invention of the mercurial gasometer and the expirator (precision instruments for measuring gas volume), ever more careful measurements of breathing were made.[30] While these new instruments were accurate and precise, the way the experiments were conducted was poor, which often led to conflicting results. This increased the rivalry between Edinburgh and Paris. To make matters worse, the units of measurement were not standardized between the two centres, as they are today. So, comparing each other's published values were fraught with errors. For gas volume, the Scots used English cubic inches, while the French used Parisian cubic inches, known today as cubic centimetres and litres. The quantity of water vapour in the air and exhaled breath was measured in either Troy grains or Troy pounds, while gas pressures and the strength of vacuums were measured against the height of mercury columns – but the columns were demarcated differently, in the UK with inches and in France with Paris lines. Eventually a consensus gradually appeared and both physicists and chemists were found to be correct: respiration or breathing was a largely mechanical and physics-based function, while respiration or metabolism was a chemical process.

How blood carried oxygen was also unknown at the time. 'Vitalist' views, such as that of the German chemist Justus Freiherr von Liebig, a prolific writer and skilled polemicist, argued that oxygen was a central force in respiration. He supported a fibrin-binding theory, in which oxygen was supposed to be bound chemically with the fibrin found in blood. This was soon disproved by fellow chemist R. Marchand, so Liebig switched to the 'protein-binding' theory originally proposed by the Dutch chemist Gerardus Mulder.[31]

As the 1800s progressed, the metaphorical fog was clearing, and many of the things we understand about breathing today were beginning to be understood as the fine structural function of the lungs was elucidated. This is when the first modern physiology textbooks began to appear and were used in medical school curricula to educate young doctors and nurses around the world. The first editions of these educational books were more conversational, and discussed current opinion rather than providing factual reviews of anatomy and physiology, as textbooks on the subject do nowadays. An early text was *Bostock's System of Physiology* (1824), which was split into subsections on areas such as the nervous system, circulation and respiration. In the first edition, the physician John Bostock acted like an editor, reviewing current opinion rather than supplying factual information. As the century progressed, physiology books became more fact-driven, with many new authors appearing. One of these was Robert Bentley Todd, who published his textbook *Cyclopedia of Anatomy and Physiology* in 1847–9. Three statements from his textbook serve to illustrate this fact-centric approach. When describing breathing's effect on the oxygen content of air: 'It would require 10,000 years, supposing the earth was peopled with 1,000,000,000 of men to produce a perceptible effect' on the atmospheric oxygen content. On respiratory disease and pollution: 'No doubt the miasmata and effluvia, which can inflict such disastrous evils on the human race, are diffused through the atmospheric air.' On the mechanics of breathing: 'Almost all men, breathe by the lower part, and the women by the upper part of their chest, and this independently of the effects of particular articles of dress!'

This widening of breathing knowledge can be illustrated by two Fellows of the Royal Society, William Allen, an English Quaker and pharmacist and William Haseldine Pepys, a scientist and descendant of Pepys the diarist. Although they both studied carbon chemistry their shared field of interest did not prevent them from making a presentation to the Royal Society on their observations on respiration on 16 June 1808. Their short four-page report is full of facts and discoveries, which they used to disprove many of the erroneous beliefs held about lung function at the time.[32] They showed that water is not made by combining oxygen and hydrogen in the lungs and that carbon dioxide concentration was raised in expiration; they measured and reported the separate volume of the left and right lungs; they measured dead space (the amount of air we do not use in each breath), the tidal volume (the breath volume) and the residual lung volume (the volume of air left in the lungs after maximal expiration); and they reported an average resting breathing rate of 19 breaths per minute. None of these facts were remarkable in themselves, but stated together they marked the beginning of the mechanistic and clinical understanding of breathing we take for granted today, and set the scene for the great epidemiologists and anthropomorphists of the late nineteenth century.

Despite research during this time being primarily supported by personal wealth, a nascent pharmacological industry was emerging. William Allen founded the pharmaceutical company Allen & Hanburys which lasted into the twentieth century, playing a significant role in the development of drugs to treat asthma. Allen & Hanburys was eventually bought out by what is today GlaxoSmithKline, who are still major suppliers of respiratory drugs globally, with a turnover of £6.9 billion in 2018.

As political revolution spread across Europe, North America and many parts of the world, the Industrial Revolution took hold in the UK. These revolutions changed the way we viewed the human spirit. Instead of looking at the individual soul, scientists and philosophers began looking outwards at the masses. The question now was not what made humans the same but what made them different. Was there something about the way Europeans breathed that accounted for their greater vitality? At this time many people believed that someone's class was predetermined by a person's heritage and biology. The next chapter tells how the epidemiology of breathing supported the justification of this misguided viewpoint.

THREE

INDUSTRY AND REVOLUTION

As the nineteenth century dawned, the world was undergoing a momentous change, with society shifting from an agriculturally based economy to an industrial one. In Great Britain, with the Industrial Revolution, the population of cities grew enormously, with a concomitant rise in population density and an equally drastic fall in the levels of sanitation. In the United States it was the Civil War (1861–5), during which the demand for healthy men of fighting age became a matter of the utmost importance, and its aftermath that changed American society and its views on civil rights and human diversity. Across Europe and the United States, two events came to shape and influence scientific and political thought for years to come: the abolition of the slave trade in America in 1865, and the publication of Charles Darwin's concept of evolution by natural selection.

While physicians and physiologists continued with their detailed mechanistic, anatomical and pathological experiments, making personal observations and using vivisection to investigate breathing control and lung function, a new avenue of enquiry blossomed in the mid-nineteenth century. A small group of scientists and physicians wondered about the range of respiratory vitality in the population at large and whether the greater prevalence of respiratory disease in the lower classes was due to inferior lungs. The invention of a single instrument engendered this new avenue of enquiry, which was to affect the lives of so many. This instrument was the spirometer, invented in the 1840s. In its initial form it was a simple medical device that accurately measured lung volume and breathing rate.[1]

U.S. President Thomas Jefferson (1743–1826) believed that slavery and in particular the prolonged labour that enslaved people were subjected to was good, as the work 'vitalized the blood' of the slaves themselves.[2] These views were based on those of Adair Crawford, a chemist and physician who in 1779 published the book *Experiments and Observations on Animal Heat*. In it he reflected the view of the ancient Greeks that breathing functioned as a mechanism to control heat. Thus, according to Jefferson, the perceived reduced lung function in black people allowed less heat to be absorbed on inspiration and to lose more heat on expiration.[3] At this time oxygen had yet to be discovered and phlogiston was thought to provide air with energy and its life-giving properties.

A New Era of Measurement

The spirometer operates on simple principles, as its function is to collect any gas or air breathed into it via a mouthpiece. In the first spirometers, expired air was collected in an inverted metal drum floating in a water bath. The drum rose in the water as it was filled by the expired breath, with the height of the risen drum being equal to the volume expelled. To standardize the test, each person was asked to inflate their lungs to the maximum by taking a big breath in, and then to empty all the air in their lungs by making an extended expiration. This requires the person to make a conscious effort to squeeze the diaphragm hard, emptying the lungs of air, at the end of expiration. It is an easy manoeuvre to do when well, but this is something we don't do often, and is painful when ill with lung disease. The breathing rate can be measured by allowing the person to breathe in through the device and recording the rate of the rise and fall of the drum. On early spirometers the drum was connected to a pen that transferred the movement of the drum onto paper. Adding known gas volumes to the drum allowed the drum excursion to be calibrated. The spirometer was a simple but elegant device that could be used outside of the laboratory.

the abdominal muscles in expiration gives rise to much higher values. This is also true of those expiratory blasts of air which are made use of in speaking, singing, coughing, and sneezing. Inasmuch as the peritoneal cavity contains no air, the individual organs are packed closely together. By closing the glottis and simultaneously contracting the diaphragm and abdominal muscles, they may be subjected to a considerable pressure, which greatly aids in the expulsion of the feces and urine. This action, which is commonly designated as the "abdominal press," also constitutes an important factor in childbirth.

Quantitative Determination of the Respired Air.—The volume of air which is taken into our lungs during a given period of time, varies with the respiratory needs of our body. Obviously, a much greater quantity of air is required when the tissues are active than when they are inactive. But while the extent and frequency of the respiratory movements may serve at any time as an indication of the intensity of the gas interchange, a direct volumetric determination of the air respired is only possible by calibration. The instrument used for this purpose is known as the *spirometer*. The one devised by Hutchinson[1] is a modified gasometer (Fig. 248). It consists of a cylindrical receptacle (*B*) filled with water, in which is suspended a second cylinder (*A*) containing air. The latter is counterbalanced by weights (*G*) in such a manner that it may be made to move with the least possible resistance. The tube (*C*) enters through the outside cylinder, and is continued upward to a level above the surface of the water in the inside compartment. If air is expired through this

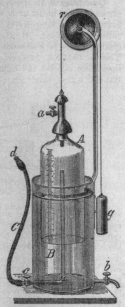

FIG. 248.—WINTRICH'S MODIFICATION OF HUTCHINSON'S SPIROMETER. (*Reichert.*)

tube, the inside cylinder rises a certain distance out of the water, while if air is inspired through it, the cylinder sinks to a lower level. The amounts of air added or subtracted in this way are indicated by a pointer upon a neighboring centimeter scale.

In order to be able to determine the volume of the air breathed in the course of a long period of time, it is necessary to know two factors, namely, the average frequency of the respiratory movements and the average volume of air respired each time. It is also possible to solve

[1] Med.-chirurg. transact., xxix, 1846, 137.

Modification of Hutchinson's spirometer by Dr Max Anton Wintrich, a German physician, 1854. It was considered easier to use: the person exhales into the tube (d) and the volume expelled could easily be read using the graduated floating dome (A). Illustration from William H. Howell, *A Text-book of Physiology for Medical Students and Physicians* (1917).

The invention of the spirometer is widely attributed to the physician John Hutchinson, who formally announced it in 1844 when presenting his initial research as a testimonial on separate occasions to the venerable London Society of Arts and the Statistical Society of London. John Hutchinson studied and practised medicine in London. Back home in Newcastle upon Tyne his father was a coal merchant, and so Hutchinson would therefore have had first-hand knowledge of coal mining and miners and their unhealthy and dusty working conditions. John Hutchinson called his device a 'spirometer', and the lung volume it measured the 'vital capacity'. He was not interested in breathing per se, but more in the relationship between lung capacity and height or stature, especially within the working population of Victorian London.

He was certainly not the first person to measure lung volume. The scientific literature describes many devices designed to do so. The Italian physiologist and mathematician Giovanni Alphonso Borelli (1608–1679) was one of the earliest persons to attempt to measure lung volume. Later the English surgeon Charles Turner Thackrah (1795–1833) during his brief lifetime working in the Midlands, used his pulmometer to assess lung function, and published his observations in 1831 in a book with the long title *The Effects of the Principal Arts, Trades and Professions, and of Civic States and Habits of Living, on Health and Longevity: with a Particular Reference to the Trades and Manufactures of Leeds, and Suggestions for the Removal of Many of the Agents, which Produce Disease, and Shorten the Duration of Life*. The book was well received at the time and describes the health problems associated with a vast range of occupations, 149 in all, and extended to 269 in his second edition of 1832.[4] During his early career Thackrah ran his own school of anatomy, and it is thought that he encouraged his students to resort to grave robbery to obtain cadavers for dissection.[5] In 1831, with the foundation of the Leeds School of Medicine, he concentrated on research. Leeds was one of the first cities in the world to undergo industrialization with the rise of the cotton mills. Thackrah was particularly critical of the dust the workers were constantly exposed to while at work, noting that 'Persons in the dusty departments are generally unhealthy. They are subject to inflammation of the lungs. The inhaled dust irritates the air-tube.'[6]

Even more concerning were the child workers who from the age of seven were exposed to this dust from half-past six in the morning until eight at night for six days a week, thirteen hours a day. This information was used by Michael Sadler in the House of Commons to establish a bill to restrict working hours. After a fifteen-year campaign the Ten Hours Act or Factory Act of 1847 was established. It was not popular with mill owners, but restricted the working hours of women and young persons (between the ages of thirteen and eighteen) in textile mills to ten hours per day. This was the first in a protracted line of legislation enacted to improve the working conditions of workers in general and eventually to outlaw child labour completely.

This period in history and the difference between Thackrah and Hutchinson reflects the switch in what medicine was largely based on, from a priori speculation to empirical observation. In 1844 Hutchinson presented his measurements of lung volumes and height collected from 1,012 males of different professions and social status, which he later increased to 2,130.[7] Hutchinson included sixty newly deceased patients in his studies. To collect measurements, he would go to the morgue and inflate the corpse with a pair of bellows until the lungs were full. He would then release the air through his spirometer; the elastic recoil of the lungs, still being present, would empty naturally.[8] This expired volume he coined the 'vital capacity', reflecting a more Darwinian view of vitality than the idea that this volume reflected health status, with a reduction in this volume being predictive of premature mortality.

Victorian sensitivities of the time discouraged the collection of lung volumes in women, as it was thought that their tight clothing might restrict the required respiratory movements. However, 26 girls were included in his reports, although his measures of chest size were made on female cadavers in the mortuary. His major discovery was that lung size was related to height irrespective of profession, class and body weight. The revolutionary aspects of Hutchinson's work were using anthropometric measures to measure health and statistically analysing the data to try and establish relationships rather than using observational data from a few case studies of patients or through animal experiments. Another revolutionary idea was to try and establish 'normality' and answer the question of what normal was, in this case the normal lung volume and breathing rate. Through statistical analysis Hutchinson could show that as height increased, so did lung volume. Today we know that lung volume depends on the size of your ribcage, which is proportional to your height or stature. When we grow as infants the various parts of our bodies grow in proportion, hence both legs reach the same size, and so on. Thus males tend to have larger lungs than females of the same height. Age also influences lung function: after reaching peak function at around 23, the lungs begin to decline, slowly at first, and then more rapidly when older age approaches, beyond sixty years. Hutchinson, although he measured the breathing rate, found the range varied widely from as slow as 6 to as fast as 40 per minute, with most men having a breathing rate in the range of 16–24.[9] This means that the amount of air we breathe in one minute (known as the minute volume) is from 6 or 7 litres per minute increasing up to around 150 litres per minute with extreme exercise. A thirty-fold increase in ventilation in a mid-distance runner may increase their ventilation to 75 litres per minute, or 4,500 litres an hour; a surprisingly small amount. An equivalent volume of water would be enough to fill a hot tub. This shows how efficient we are at breathing.

In Hutchinson's work, eighteen categories of people were described, ranging from military personnel such as sailors and First Battalion Grenadier guards to paupers and artisans, police and firemen, pugilists and wrestlers, and gentlemen. Sixty diseased cases were collected, as well as two with dwarfism and two with gigantism. He named three of these four, which may seem strange to the modern scientist, but at this time the Victorian public were interested in people of disproportionate size. Many of these people ill-treated by society ended up making a living by exhibiting themselves to the public, sometimes collectively in what later became known as freak shows, while others found sponsors. This was the case for Freeman, the American giant mentioned by Hutchinson, who originally travelled to the UK in 1840 as a prizefighter but later became an attraction. Adverts and posters stated that he could be seen working behind the bar at the Lion and Bull public house, Holborn. On another occasion he appeared in a play written for him at the Olympic Theatre.[10] He advertised his height as 7 feet 6 inches, while Hutchinson gives his height as 'upwards of 6 feet 11½ inches', where in fact he was 6 feet 9 inches tall (206 cm). After he died of tuberculosis his skeleton was donated to the Museum of the Royal College of Surgeons, London. Despite these different estimates of height, his lung capacity was measured at 464 cubic inches or 7.6 litres, an impressively large volume even today.

In 1852, following eight years of research, Hutchinson at 41 gave up his life in London, left his wife and three children behind and emigrated to Australia. The exact reasons for this are unknown; it may have been because spirometers had not become popular among physicians. Others have speculated that he had tuberculosis and the fresh air and sunshine of the tropics would cure him, a belief of the day; others think that he was suffering from alcohol abuse. Whatever the reason, he went to Melbourne, which was a just a small town then, but there was a gold rush underway, and it quickly became over-populated with speculators. Hutchinson, however, didn't seem to be interested in the gold rush. At the age of fifty he travelled to Fiji, and once there bought a large area of forest. Before he could develop his property, he caught dysentery and died. He may even have been murdered (his post-mortem showing no TB or liver disease.)[11] He was buried in an unmarked grave without leaving a will: an ignominious end.[12]

This interest in occupation was fuelled by the view that the military candidates were considered healthy and vital, representing men at the peak of fitness, while paupers and artisans were thought the opposite. People with healthy lungs did not complain of breathlessness and unobstructed breathing was considered a sign of good health, especially in the polluted and smoke-filled cities of industrialized Europe. Eventually the spirometer was adopted by scientists and physicians around the world. As a precision instrument it could be manufactured easily. A plethora of makers appeared, around 27 by the end of the century, and at around £5 10s. it was not too expensive for individual physicians to purchase.[13]

In the mid-eighteenth century research into breathing and lung function was sparse in the USA, but this was to change after the four years of the American Civil War (1861–5), when eleven southern states formed the Confederacy and attacked the remaining largely northern states, the Union. The causes of the war were complex but centred around the wish to ban slavery in the USA; the Confederate states were against these moves. An early defeat of the Union army at the Battle of Bull Run in July 1861 led to President Abraham Lincoln creating a government body to oversee the relief efforts and sanitary conditions of the army. As the war progressed, this body, the United States Sanitary Commission, decided to do a survey of social and physical characteristics of the Union Army. The survey was started by General Secretary Frederick Law Olmsted, an architect by profession, but was continued in 1864 by Benjamin Apthorp Gould, an esteemed Boston astronomer. Gould, keen to collect the best data he could, planned to measure stature, complexion, proportions of the body and head, weight, respiratory rate and pulse, and pulmonary capacity. His survey of 21,752 soldiers was published as *Investigations in the Military and Anthropological Statistics of American Soldiers* in 1869. Instead of treating the soldiers as a homogenous group, Gould categorized his data by nativity, age and race, the last in categories such as white, black, 'mulatto' (or mixed race) and 'Indian'. Gould reported lung function in 18,580 white personnel and 511 Native Americans. The white soldiers had a mean lung capacity of 185 cubic inches or 3.0 litres, while the 2,661 black and mixed-race soldiers had a volume of 161 cubic inches or 2.6 litres. The breathing data showed a similar discrepancy, with the white population breathing an average rate of 17 breaths per minute and the black soldiers faster at 18. It was noted that the black soldiers were measured in the South, where it was warmer. Most of the black soldiers would have previously been enslaved Southern plantation workers and had suffered from poor living conditions before joining the Union Army. They had a higher mortality rate and received worse medical care and living conditions than their contemporary white colleagues, so consequently were more likely to suffer from respiratory disease. Despite these obvious differences in living conditions, the differences in breathing were used to confirm the common view held by the white population at the time that blacks were biologically inferior.

A later study by the Bureau of the War Department which included a million soldiers and was conducted by the chief medical officer Jedediah H. Baxter was published in tabular form in 1875 in two volumes under the title *Statistics, Medical and Anthropological, of the Provost-Marshall-General's Bureau, Derived from Records of the Examination for Military Service in the Armies of the United States during the Late War of the Rebellion of Over a Million Recruits, Drafted Men, Substitutes and Enrolled Men.* Compiled under the Direction of the Secretary of War. This huge study did not use spirometry but instead measured chest circumference and expansion on breathing. The study found no difference between the white European nationalities and black recruits. This data was used to argue for the fitness of African Americans to be good soldiers, as a low vital capacity was considered a sign of lower vitality. The New Orleans historian, ex-plantation owner and Confederate sympathizer Charles Gayarré wrote: 'Should the black man die out in the end, as he probably will, of weak lungs and from the want of congenial air in the more elevated region to which he has been raised, and to which he cannot be acclimated, let it not be recorded that it is due to bad treatment on our part.'[14]

During the latter half of the century many physicians promoted the notion that reduced lung capacity and predisposition to respiratory disease marked blacks as inferior.[15] This notion that the European lung volumes constituted the benchmark of normal lung function was extended to the end of the twentieth century. The inequalities in access to good nutrition and healthcare were not considered to be the probable cause of these differences. To the Victorians, the reason was biological inferiority. Finding physical differences between the classes and races helped reinforce white European supremacy, along with the views of gentlemanly superiority over the working majority. In the USA it drove the health and exercise movement and eventually fed into the idea of eugenics.

Spirometry was considered an important anthropometric measure, as lung size could be predicted from a person's height, providing a view of what was normal. This allowed those who were screening recruits or members of the public to define the healthy lung size, which was equated with vitality. A 'normal' value derived mainly from males who were Anglo-Saxon in origin led, particularly in the USA, to comparisons between 'vitality' and race. The data was used politically to inform U.S. policy and commercially to determine the cost of life insurance. However, in Europe, spirometry was applied only to professions and not races, so although it tended to split the population class-wise, its impact on society was small, since class division was common already.

Understanding Respiratory Disease

In the Victorian era, one common respiratory disease was tuberculosis (TB). Although it was infectious, its cause was uncertain. It was also known by the names phthisis (named after the Greek god of decay, the word means 'dwindling' or 'wasting away') and consumption, as the final stages were characterized by a progressive wasting of the body and a persistent cough, often accompanied by bloody expectorant and night sweats. The modern name was coined in 1882 when the German physician and microbiologist Robert Heinrich Hermann Koch discovered that it was the bacteria *Mycobacterium tuberculosis* that was the causative agent. TB infection follows poverty and spreads easily, especially in places where population density is high. The more communal the living

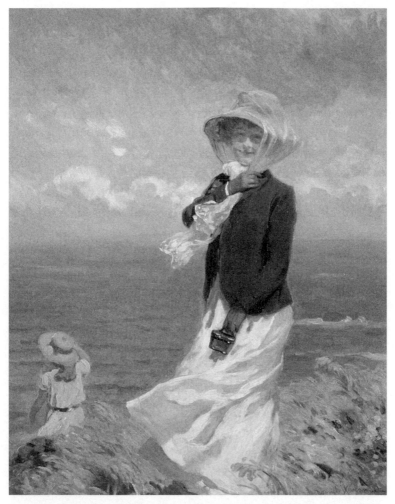

Daniel Hernández (1856–1932), *A Windy Day*, oil on canvas. People with
TB were recommended to leave urban areas and move where the air was
considered cleaner: to the coast, a warmer climate or higher altitude.

conditions the higher the rate. In the nineteenth century it was
said that worldwide 1 in 7 deaths were due to TB. The UK figures
for the decade 1881–90 show that out of a total of 5,244,771 deaths,
589,390 were due to TB, around 1 in 11.[16] By 1939, in North America,
TB mortality was 61,000 (42 per 100,000 of the population); in
Europe it was higher, a total of 442,000–522,000 deaths (around
110–200 per 100,000 of the population). Today, with vaccination
and antibiotics, TB is less common in the UK. In 2018 there were

5,900 cases (9 per 100,000 of the population) with around 282 deaths in 2012 (0.4 per 100,000 of the population). In other parts of the world the story is different, with South Africa suffering the highest rates and the USA the lowest. It is still one of the world's top ten most deadly diseases and is the leading cause of deaths that are due to a single infectious agent. There are now around 1.7 billion people in the world who are infected with *mycobacterium tuberculosis* but are free of symptoms.[17] In 2018 around 1.5 million people died from TB.

In the nineteenth century a widely advocated treatment was fresh air, meaning unpolluted air. Those who could afford to often left the polluted cities and moved to rural areas or abroad to places where either the climate was warm and dry, such as in the Mediterranean, or the air was considered pure, such as in the Alps in Europe and the Adirondacks in the USA. Later the creation of TB sanatoriums allowed anyone with TB to live in (often for months) and breathe as much fresh air as possible. These sanatoriums were located in isolated locations away from population centres and deliberately placed to receive fresh winds and weather. Thus TB sufferers left their families and lives behind. Sanatoriums began to disappear after the 1950s when antibiotic treatment became available.

When town air was still considered fresh air, other treatment advice was offered, from the dangerous and false, such as mustard plasters (which blister the skin) and tonics (containing mostly alcohol), to lifestyle changes. Those with TB were thought to have weak lungs and therefore one way to keep healthy was to maintain good breathing.

Influential physiology textbooks of the time not only provided a description of the anatomy and physiology of the lungs but advice on how to remain healthy and avoid TB and bronchitis. An influential text by father and son Edward Hitchcock and Edward Hitchcock Jr, *Elementary Anatomy and Physiology, for Colleges, Academies and Other Schools* (1860), advocated standing with the chest forward and sleeping with the window open at night to ensure that the maximum amount of fresh air is breathed. The advice continues, stating that whatever compresses the chest greatly tends to bring on diseases of the chest. Thus men should not wear shawls,

> for that the wearing of shawls by gentlemen, in as much as it requires a drawing forward of the shoulders to make them thoroughly cover the body, compresses the lungs, and therefore is highly injurious. Moreover, it makes a person round shouldered, and thus gives the appearance of premature old age.

If shawls were bad, then scarves and neckties were worse, 'For tight cravats and neckcloths are sure to obstruct the proper function of this organ [larynx], and bring on irritation, which may end in bronchitis or consumption.'

Even more bizarre advice can be found in a popular book of the time written by Diocletian Lewis of Boston, Massachusetts, called *Weak Lungs and How to Make Them Strong; or, Diseases of the Organs of the Chest with Their Home Treatment by the Movement Cure* (1864). The three-hundred-page book is full of advice on how to avoid contracting consumption, by methods such as wearing wool instead of linen. It is full of such bizarre advice that it is worth quoting. For example, on footwear Lewis offers this advice:

> As the health of the feet has much to do with the health of the lungs, I submit a suggestion or two. First, the sole should be broad and strong, and the heels broad and long. The width of the sole is most important. Nothing can be more absurd and crueler than the present narrow soles. The broad-toed boots and shoes are physiological.

He believed women's shoes to be too narrow. Lewis had even more extreme views about the link between hair and consumption:

> The management of our hair has much to do with the health of the respiratory apparatus. Cutting it short behind,

and thus exposing the upper part of the spine to the changes of the atmosphere, exerts an injurious influence upon the larynx and its contained vocal apparatus. The present fashion among women, of hanging the hair in a net on the back of the neck, is not only physiological, but, in my opinion, in excellent taste.

His advice continues:

> Shaving off the beard exposes the larynx and trachea. If it be asked why man needs this protection more than women, I reply, that the larynx, which, in women, is buried in and surrounded by the soft parts, is in man, prominent and exposed; and if the neck be nude, greatly exposed to atmospheric influences. But a better reason is this: – God contrived the beard for man's neck. It is His plan that man should wear this protection over the throat. In the light of this evident purpose of the Creator.

Exercise was another important factor, especially breathing exercises, and here he recommended starting all exercise with a warm-up using the spirometer, his reasoning being that 'Its use opens all the air cells, and fully prepares the lungs for those deep inspirations, which are so important to the most profitable muscular training.' Alternatively, if the consumptive person did not possess a spirometer, 'the same result may be reached to a considerable extent by filling the lungs as full as possible, and blowing, holding the hand over the mouth so that no air can escape.'

The gymnastic exercises recommended were lifting bar bells and clubs and various stretching manoeuvres. Many required working against another person's hold or restraint: 'In many of the exercises, you have one or two assistants. These should be gentle and patient persons. Your servant, if you have one, will generally prove the best assistant. He or she does not feel at liberty to wrestle with you but will quietly follow your instructions.'

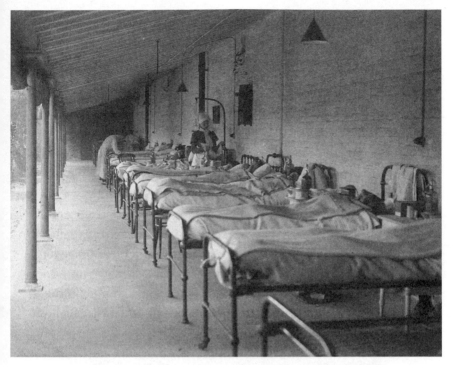

Open-air tuberculosis ward during the First World War, at the Royal Hospital Haslar, Gosport, England, which housed military personnel since the 1700s. Several of the patients are still wearing their regimental berets.

As soon as your exercises are finished, you must dress yourself warmly, and lie down for an hour or two, to sleep, if possible. This will double the good effects of the exercise. Any hurry or flurry about the patient is unfavourable. Let all be done in quietness and cheerfulness.

Lewis may have had an influential personality – he was a temperance leader, a preacher, a feminist, a social reformer and a food/health faddist – but he was not a doctor. He did use the title and sometimes practised illegally. This could explain his exaggerated links between the body form and function and TB. One thing that is central to his advice is that deep breathing was considered vital in maintaining healthy lungs.

Applied Spirometry

The spirometer's measure of vital lung capacity was considered a sound indicator of health when screening potential military recruits, so it is no surprise that it was used to assess health in other groups. Young male university graduates were an obvious choice. This view corresponded with the fashion, particularly prevalent in the USA, for collegiate exercise programmes. Gymnasiums were added to university campuses in the USA and around the world. By the 1880s virtually every major American university and some European universities had their own gymnasiums and it became compulsory for students to exercise daily or risk being expelled. Lung vital capacity was measured regularly and breathing exercises or 'lung gymnastics' were advocated by many gym trainers. Deep breathing for several minutes was supposed to stimulate respiration, leading to mental stimulation, which in turn dispelled feelings of sluggishness or sleepiness.[18]

This was the industrial age, so soon inventors began to advocate the use of breathing machines. These machines were the forefathers of the machines we find in gyms today. Modern exercise machines are designed to provide cardiovascular exercise or improve muscle strength and mass by allowing the exerciser to lift weights, run on a treadmill or cycle on a fixed cycle or ergometer. Using these running and cycling machines (and their derivatives, such as skiing and rowing) will increase breathing rate and depth. The early pioneers of these mechanical exercise machines were using them to promote well-being by 'mechanotherapy'. One of the earliest pioneers was the Swedish physician Jonas Gustav Wilhelm Zander, who founded the Zander Institute first in Stockholm in the 1890s and then later in New York, and across the USA by the early 1900s. A lot of his machines were brutal, as the electrically powered paddles and pedals were not very refined. By the 1930s the machines became more developed and began to resemble the exercise machines we are used to seeing today.

One such device was 'The Tower', designed by Zander specifically to exercise respiratory movements.[19] The device clamps both

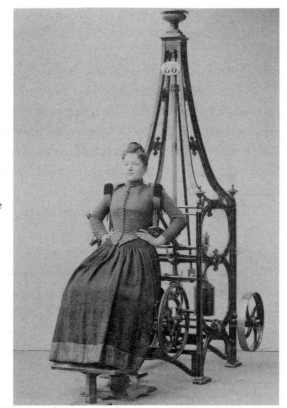

'The Tower' to aid respiratory movements: an exercise machine designed by Dr Gustav Zander. The shoulders are held firmly, while pressure is applied to the back. Illustration from Alfred Levertin, *Dr G. Zander's Medico-mechanische Gymnastik* (1892).

the shoulders back, keeping them still while the machine applies positive pressure rhythmically to the mid-back. The applied pressure forces the person to breathe out. Another breathing machine, called the Quarter Circle, allows the person to lift weights while lying on their back on a curved board; another was Taylor's Spinal Assistant, which stretched the person by suspending them by their arms, with their body weight being supported on their side (laterally), or while lying on their front or back. Today these would be considered instruments of torture, not exercise.

The advent of the First World War brought the assessment of lung function to the fore again, particularly with the foundation in 1918 of the Royal Air Force (RAF) in Great Britain. As the Air Force gained greater and greater strategic power, pilots' health became paramount. The effects of altitude or high flying meant that a greater understanding of oxygen deprivation was needed. Pilot deaths had previously been put down to lack of physical fitness or carelessness. While assessing lung function was important, what was more important was the realization that the deaths were due to the pilots blacking out from hypoxia (oxygen deprivation at altitude). This link between function and performance again reinforced the notion that breathing and vital capacity were an indicator of potential performance. The need to regulate oxygen supply and the effects of hypoxia drove the development of innovative technology. At the RAF this drive was led by Georges Dreyer, a physician and scientist of Danish origin.

The widespread application of spirometry soon pointed to its usefulness as a tool for screening respiratory health. Following the work begun by Hutchinson, it was now known that a person's lung function could be predicted from their age, height and gender. Those who benefited the most from this were miners. From just after the First World War to the 1930s, coal was the major fuel driving industry, transport and domestic heating. In the UK around 250 million tonnes a year of coal was mined, and at its peak in the 1920s the industry employed 1,191,000 miners. During the early twentieth century the miners worked long shifts and would spend many hours a day working underground. The mines were dusty places full of both coal and rock dust. The carbonaceous coal dust was thought to be inert and therefore not a health issue. Thus when miners developed occupational lung diseases, other causes were sought. Miners' lung disease was thought to be caused by the silica from the rock dust, which resulted in silicosis. Gradually evidence began to accumulate that this wasn't the case, and soon coal dust was confirmed to be the cause of lung disease in many miners (who often smoked tobacco as well). This condition was called pneumoconiosis (from the Greek *konis*, meaning 'dust'). Breathing coal dust for many years led to lung scarring, which takes many years of exposure before it becomes apparent. A person with pneumoconiosis becomes breathless and suffers a dry cough. Oxygen cannot cross into the blood as easily as it should because the lungs are inflamed and scarred.

After the Second World War, the coal miners became unionized. In the UK the National Union of Mineworkers (formed in 1945) became interested in their members' health. It was quickly realized that spirometry could be used as a screening tool for pneumoconiosis. Thus the detection of decline in lung function was a useful aid in the creation of a national coal industry pneumoconiosis compensation scheme, funded by the government. In mining areas, the unions and the legal profession began to represent claimants who were unable to work due to pneumoconiosis. The need for lung-function testing by the NHS created extra demand on health services, as doctors had to confirm that the disease was present. Today, this legacy continues: exposure risk is underwritten by insurance companies and it is the cornerstone of occupational health that any employee who works in a dusty environment needs to have their lung function monitored by undergoing regular (annual) spirometry.

In southern Africa gold and diamond mining was another source of occupational lung disease. In 1886 gold was discovered in the region, resulting in a gold rush. Many miners came from Cornwall and Devon, as the mining of tin and copper there had become less profitable. The European miners were supported by a large number of local migrant workers and, later, indentured Chinese workers. By 1910 there were around 10,000 Europeans and 120,000 black miners working in 87 pits who had by then extracted millions of tons of gold. The Cornish miners typically worked for five years in the mines before returning home, and it was in these returning miners that the first signs of silicosis were noticed. The death rate was significant enough for a Royal Commission to be set up to investigate under the leadership of the Scottish physiologist John Scott Haldane (1860–1936). The disease was called 'miners' phthisis', as it was at first thought to be mining-induced TB. Its prevalence in rock drillers was high and could not be ignored, not even by mine owners.

A health compensation scheme was established for the affected miners. Those of European origin would be compensated with a monthly allowance, while in black miners silicosis was treated as an injury and therefore they received a single lump-sum payment. The publication of the findings on the extent and prevention of coal pneumoconiosis in the 1950s in the clinical literature inspired clinicians in southern Africa to research further. It was only then that the full extent of mining on breathing and lung disease was realized. Although the government set about regulating exposure to dust, the dichotomous treatment of the miners in South Africa did not change until apartheid was dismantled in 1994.[20]

It can be seen that the invention of the spirometer had an important cultural impact beyond its original function of quantifying the differences in breathing and lung vitality between professions and classes in Victorian London. The simple spirometer has made its mark in 'national and social worlds': biomedicine, life insurance, the culture of physical exercise, the military, philanthropy, eugenics, anthropometry and workers' compensation systems.[21]

Breathing in the Twentieth Century

The twentieth century began with two hundred years of accumulated knowledge on breathing. The gross anatomical structure of the lungs was known, the mechanics of breathing were well understood and the link between circulation and the carriage of oxygen in the blood had been clarified. Or so everyone thought. Unbeknown to the world, a revolution in our understanding was about to be realized. With advances in technology came cleverer and more detailed studies. Attention to the fine microstructure of the lungs and cardiovascular system provided new insights into breathing.

However, the association between breathing and body heat had not been resolved. This is reflected in the idea of spontaneous human combustion, a disputed condition in which the body bursts into flames, causing death. The idea was popularized by the English novelist Charles Dickens in his novel *Bleak House* (1852–3), where Mr Krook, a scruffy and alcoholic landlord, is alone in his parlour drinking when he bursts into flames. A passer-by in the street, a Mr Snagsby, smells 'chops being grilled', while the tenants upstairs comment on rising soot and the formation of a 'thick yellow liquor'. Dickens's readers accepted spontaneous combustion as fact, but many in the scientific and medical community criticized him, saying that he was pandering to superstition. Dickens stood his ground and stated that he had personally attended dozens of coroner's inquests of people who had died this way.

Even as recently as 2011 an Irish coroner, Ciaran McLoughlin, recorded an unexplained death as due to spontaneous combustion: 76-year-old Michael Flaherty, who was found burnt to death next to his fireplace. While it was not suggested that his body burst into flames of its own accord, there was no external source of ignition identified.

Oxygen is highly reactive and can be used with hydrogen as a rocket fuel, so when we breathe it in such copious quantities, why do we not burst into flames? This paradox has only been recently solved by chemists from the USA; it seems that in the body, oxygen behaves differently in the presence of hydrogen. In the body oxygen and hydrogen do not react explosively. This creates oxygen free radicals, which have a bad press, as they have been shown to damage cells and DNA, but may be essential in protecting the body against excess combustion.

The Scottish physiologist John Scott Haldane made great contributions to our understanding of breathing. He was keen to improve public health, as little attention was being paid to ill health caused by exposure to poisonous atmospheres in mines. Haldane, through self-experimentation, showed that normal viated air (a mixture of room air and expired air) did not contain any peculiar organic compounds and that expired air just contained more carbon dioxide and water than inspired air. The toxic culprit in most cases was carbon monoxide, CO, which is created when burning carbonaceous material such as coal and tobacco. If this is done in a confined, ill-ventilated place, toxic levels (around 2 per cent) can be reached quickly and insidiously. Haldane also investigated the effects of anoxia (lack of oxygen) on breathing.

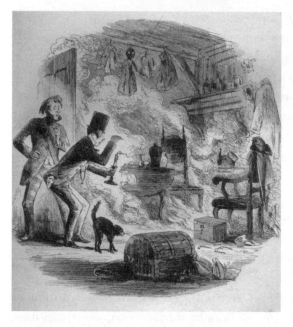

After following a burning smell in the house, Mr Guppy and Tony Jobling, alias Mr Weevle, observe a cat snarling at a pile of white ashes. The ashes are the remains of the landlord Mr Crook, who has undergone a fiery death of 'Spontaneous Combustion, and none other of all the deaths that can be died.' Illustration by Phiz for Charles Dickens, *Bleak House* (1852-3).

These studies allowed him to firmly link ill health and death to bad ventilation in rooms with coal fires, poorly ventilated mineshafts or railway tunnels. Haldane investigated the way oxygen and the carbonaceous gases (CO_2 and CO) were carried in the blood.

Alveolar oxygen is taken up into the blood where it binds to a red pigmented protein called haemoglobin. Each haemoglobin molecule in mammals has evolved to present four iron atoms. Each iron atom can reversibly bind oxygen atoms. Blood is red because of this haemoglobin and the red is imparted by the iron-oxygen compound. The cells filled with haemoglobin are called erythrocytes (or red blood cells). Each red blood cell contains roughly 270 million haemoglobin molecules, and there are on average 20-30 trillion red blood cells in the average adult. Haemoglobin can also carry a small amount of carbon dioxide. Haldane showed that haemoglobin's ability to do this was altered by oxygen levels. This is known as the Haldane effect.

There were still discoveries yet to be made about the air we breathe. Lord Rayleigh (born John William Strutt, 1842-1919), despite working for many years measuring the amount of oxygen and nitrogen in air, was unable, like other scientists, to agree upon their exact proportions, which seemed to differ depending on the method used to prepare the gases. It wasn't until he began working with the Scottish chemist Sir William Ramsey (1852–1916) that this discrepancy was resolved with the discovery that it was due to an impurity: an extra inactive gas and new element, which they called argon, symbol Ar (from the Greek *aergon*, meaning 'inert' or 'lazy'). The pair announced their discovery to the world in 1894. The new gas had physical and chemical properties that did not fit in with the other elements known at the time, nor did it fit anywhere in the periodic table. This led other chemists to doubt whether argon existed or if it was even an element. This did not deter Ramsey, who continued his studies and later went on to define other elemental gases: helium (He), and then a whole family of helium-like gases, krypton (Kr, Greek: *krypos*, 'hidden'), xenon (Xe, Greek: *xenos*, 'stranger'), neon (Ne, Greek: *neos*, 'new') and eventually radioactive radon (Ra). Argon fits between neon and krypton in the series.

In 1904 Rayleigh received the Nobel Prize in Physics for this discovery, while Ramsey received the Nobel Prize in Chemistry 'in recognition of his services in the discovery of inert gaseous elements in the air'. Ramsey died of nasal cancer, which most likely resulted from spending a life sniffing noxious gases. The gases were eventually called the noble gases and now occupy their own column and group (18) in the periodic table. They gained this soubriquet from the belief that they did not react with other elements.

The air we breathe contains exceedingly small amounts of xenon, of which there are nine forms or isotopes. While 80 per cent of this xenon is of terrestrial origin, around 20 per cent comes from outer space and has been delivered to Earth in colliding comets.[22] The majority of the alien xenon arrived 3.6 billion years ago when the Earth and moon underwent an intense bombardment of comets. This discovery was made only recently by the ESA Rosetta mission, which visited the comet 67P/Churyumov-Gerasimenko in 2014–16. The Rosetta craft found that the comet contained lots of the unearthly xenon isotope.

At the end of the nineteenth century and in the early twentieth century, many of the investigations into breathing shifted to the European continent, namely Austria, Denmark and Germany. Before the Great War it was easy to travel around Europe, and scientists from all scientific disciplines began to meet at international congresses. This is where the history of breathing passes to the biochemists and physiologists, who used their skills to investigate breathing at the molecular and cellular level and made new discoveries. The most vexing question at the time was: how did the two gases, oxygen and carbon dioxide, pass between the air, blood and tissues? Careful measurements by different researchers provided conflicting results.

Two theories predominated; one school of thought believed that oxygen exchange from the air to blood relied on diffusion

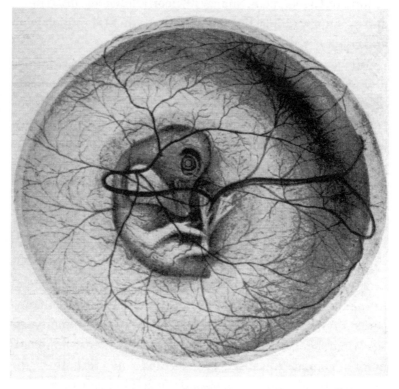

Goose embryo in its shell, showing the allantois and its diffuse vessels. The shell is sufficiently porous to allow air to diffuse in, letting the embryo respire. Illustration by William Bell, 1793.

alone, a natural physical process. With diffusion oxygen simply passes down a concentration gradient (that is, moves outwards from an area of high concentration to an area of low concentration), thus crossing the alveolar membrane into the blood, with oxygen levels in the alveoli being higher than in the blood, especially during inspiration of fresh air. The second theory posited that energy was needed to actively transport oxygen from the lung across the alveolar membrane into the blood. Haldane believed this active secretion hypothesis. His measurements of blood oxygen levels suggested that the oxygen content of arterial blood in the lungs was higher than the amount in the air, so diffusion was not possible and therefore oxygen must be actively transported from the alveoli and secreted into the blood. This view was supported by others, including the prominent Danish physiologist Christian Harald Lauritz Peter Emil Bohr, who worked in Copenhagen and corresponded regularly with Haldane. They often visited each other's laboratories. Bohr's main contribution to our understanding of breathing is through his work on the transport of oxygen in the blood. Through careful experimentation he showed that when oxygen bound to haemoglobin in the red blood cells, it did so in an S-shaped fashion and not a simple linear, one-for-one fashion. An interaction between the group of four iron atoms on each haemoglobin molecule is responsible. An S-shaped curve means that the uptake of oxygen into the blood cells occurs at different rates depending on the amount of oxygen already in the blood, so when blood oxygen levels are low, as when blood enters the lungs, many of the iron atoms are unoccupied by oxygen and are free to absorb oxygen more easily. When the iron sites are full, the rate of oxygen uptake slows. He went on to show how the S-shape was influenced by carbon dioxide; this is now known as the Bohr effect.[23] We now know this S-shape or sigmoid shape is due to the molecular structure of the haemoglobin molecule and the conditions of the gel (cytoplasm) surrounding them within the red cell, which is especially important under different environmental conditions, whether it be on the top of a mountain or within a developing foetus in the womb.

Not everyone accepted Bohr and Haldane's excretion view. One 'diffusionist' was a student of Bohr's, Schack August Steenberg Krogh, a Dane, who later became Professor of Zoophysiology at the University of Copenhagen from 1916 to 1945. Krogh began working with Bohr in 1897 as a postgraduate student; his project was to improve the precision of arterial blood oxygen content measurements. Through careful study he and his assistant, Marie Jørgensen, a physician, became convinced that the diffusion route was enough to drive oxygen transport. In 1905 he married Marie. As husband and wife, they worked quietly together trying to provide supporting evidence backing Bohr's theory. They failed and the opposite happened: the harder they tried to prove him right, with ever more detailed experiments, the more the evidence pointed to Bohr being wrong. They finally broke their silence in 1910 when they published their results. A publication in 1909 by Bohr advocating the oxygen secretion theory had forced their hand.[24] They published a series of seven papers on the subject, all in the same journal, the *Skandinavisches Archiv fur Physiologie*. These papers were later nicknamed the 'Seven Devils' by August Krogh.[25]

The Kroghs' first paper on the subject, simply titled 'On the Tensions of Gases in the Arterial Blood', showed that the blood oxygen levels in the pulmonary artery were lower than the oxygen levels in the air inside the lungs, enough to allow diffusion alone to drive oxygen.[26] The final two of the seven papers specifically point out that Bohr was wrong. (Bohr refused to believe this and did not change his mind until his sudden early death in February 1911, aged 56.) Bohr had two sons, Niels, the physicist who won the Nobel Prize in Physics in 1922, and Harald, who became a mathematician. Neils Bohr's son, Aage, also received a Nobel Prize in Physics in 1975, quite an impressive achievement for one family.

One way to solve this conflict would be to measure blood oxygen content at altitude, so an expedition to high altitude was considered. The reasoning behind this is that as the oxygen pressure at altitude is lower than at sea level, this would exaggerate any differences between the alveolar and blood oxygen levels. In the end several expeditions were required, each at an ever-increasing altitude. The first expedition was in 1910, led by Joseph Barcroft, a British high-altitude physiologist, who ascended to the 3,718-metre (12,198 ft) volcanic peak of Mount Teide, Tenerife, in the Canary Islands; the second, in 1911, was by Haldane, Douglas, Henderson and Schneider, to the 4,302-metre (14,115 ft) Pikes Peak in the Rocky Mountains of Colorado. In the same year Barcroft also visited Monte Rosa in the Italian Alps, Europe's second highest mountain at 4,634 metres (15,203 ft). The data collected during these expeditions did not help with the oxygen secretion theory, and even Haldane began to doubt its correctness.

The final blows came from two directions: from Marie Krogh in 1915 and a further high-altitude expedition in 1921–2. In 1915 Marie Krogh published the work for her doctoral thesis in a paper with the short title 'The Diffusion of Gases through the Lungs of Man'. She showed how carbon monoxide crossed from the lungs into the blood by diffusion without the need for active transport. The 1921 expedition was led again by Joseph Barcroft, to the city of Cerro de Pasco, a silver-mining area in the Peruvian Andes at an elevation of 4,330 metres (14,210 ft). This high-altitude town was linked by rail, so upon arriving in Cerro de Pasco they were able to convert their railway carriage into a fully functioning laboratory. Despite these fine laboratory facilities, the team of eight still could not provide any supporting evidence for the secretion theory. Like Bohr, however, Haldane remained convinced until his death in 1936.

August Krogh received the 1920 Nobel Prize in Medicine or Physiology for his work on oxygen diffusion in muscles rather than lungs. He retired from his professorship in 1946 at the age of 72. After developing diabetes, Marie, along with August and Hans Christian Hagedorn, started a pharmaceutical company, Novo Nordisk, which supplied the Scandinavian countries with insulin. Marie died of breast cancer in 1943. Novo Nordisk is still in existence and in 2017 employed around 43,000 people, with an annual revenue of 112 billion Danish krone (around £13.5 billion).

The last major advances in our understanding of breathing are to be found in the blood. It was observed early that blood

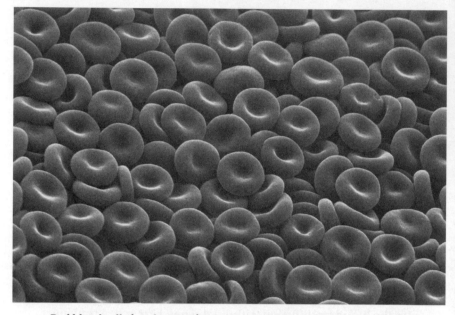

Red blood cells (erythrocytes) carry oxygen and their unique biconcave shape allows them to squeeze through narrow capillaries and to present a large surface area for gas exchange. Electromicrograph by Annie Cavanagh, n.d.

colour differed: in the veins it is a burgundy colour, in the arteries scarlet. It was some time before this colour difference was associated with the oxygen we breathe. The scarlet colour reflects oxygen binding to the four iron atoms presented by the protein molecule haemoglobin; the burgundy colour reflects unbound haemoglobin, or deoxygenated blood, typically venous blood. In order to chemically analyse the function of this complex oxygen-carrying protein it needed to be crystallized. This was done by 1850 using the blood of squirrels and other animals.[27] The iron content of blood had been known since the eighteenth century, and this portion of the blood was then termed 'haematin'. It wasn't until 1862 that the term 'haemoglobin' (the American spelling is hemoglobin) was coined by the German chemist Felix Hoppe-Seyler. Hoppe-Seyler performed a lot of spectroscopy using crystallized haemoglobin and showed how the molecule changed structurally with oxygen binding. Along with the mathematician and physicist George Gabriel Stokes, he noted that there are two forms or oxidation states, which Stokes called 'scarlet cruorine' and 'purple cruorine'.[28] Hoppe-Seyler coined the terms in common use today: 'oxyhaemoglobin' and 'deoxyhaemoglobin' for the scarlet and purple forms, respectively. At this time, the German chemist Gustav von Hüfner proved that oxygen bound to the haemoglobin molecule. Then, over the next hundred years, the size of the haemoglobin molecule was elucidated and found to consist of around 580 amino acids. The protein was made of smaller units called globulins, four in all, each with its own iron-containing carbon-ring-structure compound called a porphyrin. Thus a shortage of elemental iron in our bodies can have serious effects on our breathing; if we become anaemic (iron deficient), then we can feel breathless and lethargic through lack of haemoglobin and fewer oxygen-carrying sites.

The next major discovery awaited the Austrian chemist Max Ferdinand Perutz, working with his colleague at the University of Cambridge, the biochemist John Kendrew. Perutz left Austria following the Anschluss in 1938. Settling in Cambridge, he began working with Lawrence Bragg, a Nobel Prize winner and the director of the Cavendish Laboratory, starting his long journey towards elucidating the three-dimensional structure of haemoglobin. X-ray crystallography was used to define the structure of proteins and more famously the structure of the double helix of DNA. It took until 1959 to finally define the structure of haemoglobin. In 1962 Perutz and Kendrew received the Nobel Prize in Chemistry for their studies on finding the structure of haemoglobin.

In the twentieth century research into the role of breathing and associated pathologies attracted several Nobel Prizes. In 1905 the German bacteriologist Robert Koch received the prize in Physiology or Medicine for his work on tuberculosis; August Krogh won it in 1920; Otto Meyerhof received the prize in Physiology or Medicine for his work on oxygen metabolism in 1922. In 1931 another Otto, the German biochemist Otto Heinrich Warburg, received the prize in Physiology or Medicine for his work on cellular oxygen consumption and the respiratory enzymes that cells contain. The following year, 1932, Sir Charles Sherrington and

Edgar Adrian received the prize in Physiology or Medicine for their discoveries regarding the function of neurons, which involved experiments on goldfish breathing. Next, in 1938, the Belgian physiologist Corneille Heymans received the prize in Physiology and Medicine, on the sensing mechanisms that control breathing. The twenty-first century is still young but the 2019 prize in Physiology or Medicine went to William G. Kaelin Jr, Sir Peter J. Ratcliffe and Gregg L. Semenza for their discoveries of how cells sense and adapt to oxygen availability.

THE TECHNOLOGICAL ADVANCES that emerged from the global industrialization of society during the eighteenth century led to new ways of measuring breathing. The mass production of these measuring devices, such as the spirometer, allowed measurements to be made en masse, founding the discipline of epidemiology. Simple to use, the spirometer allowed questions to be asked of populations and society, such as 'What is normal function?' and 'How do we define abnormal?' The accompanying revolution in chemistry and physics allowed close analysis of the physiology of breathing, and for its mechanism to be measured with ever-greater precision and accuracy. Through these advances in medicine and science we not only learnt how we breathe, but began to discover something else: to stay healthy, we need to breathe clean, fresh air. With industrialization and advancing technology came unprecedented air pollution, smog and increased respiratory-associated mortality.

FOUR

MIASMA AND BAD AIR

W hile our understanding of breathing was revealed bit by bit through careful investigation, the idea that the air we breathe is always the same, and the notion that air quality is paramount to good health, became clear to society in general and governments in particular. Foul air had long been considered evil and associated with spirits, witchcraft and mysterious sprites. Typically, respiratory ill health was associated with areas of stagnant and polluted waters around mires, marshes and bogs. Humankind's role in maintaining air quality became apparent only with the advent of the Industrial Revolution.

Foul Air

For many centuries it was accepted that breathing and disease were intimately connected. Breathing air that was too hot, cold, dry or wet was thought to be the cause of many diseases and fevers. One term for this bad air was miasma. In ancient Greek the word 'miasma' is derived from the verb *miaino*, which means to stain, rather like a bloodstain.[1] The word did not appear in a medical context until the fifth century BC, after which it was used to denote air that contained contagious disease. Hippocrates wrote in his treatise on the nature of man that disease came 'from the air we breathe in to live'. In his treatise *Breaths*, he states that the major cause of pestilential disease is the inhalation or air and that the air is polluted with odours originating from the putrefaction of uncremated cadavers or fumes from swamps or lakes during the summer.[2]

The Roman physician Galen built on this idea and spoke of the danger of living with those affected by pestilence as these people exhale polluted air.[3] This malevolent and simple view of bad air was accepted unquestioned until the nineteenth century. The general belief that bad air was influenced by the climate and seasons dominated thinking and few people tried to do anything about removing this air. However, one of the earliest attempts to improve public health by recognizing how to prevent the effects of bad air was made by the English reverend and physiologist Stephen Hales (1677–1761), who, in the 1740s, proposed installing giant ventilators to circulate air around ships' decks, prisons and hospitals, where death from overcrowding was common. The idea of 'hygienic ventilation' was born.

Prominent anti-miasmatists of the nineteenth century included the social reformer Edwin Chadwick, who helped improve the Poor Laws and instigate major reforms in urban sanitation and public health, and nurse Florence Nightingale, who continued with the belief that disease was created and carried by air derived from rotting organic material, sewage and polluted water. Now the source of the foul air was the overcrowded populace in city slums. Marshes and bogs were no longer considered a major source as those near cities had been drained and those remaining were located a long way away from the centres of population.

Florence Nightingale's *Notes on Nursing* (1859) gives pages and pages of advice on how pure air is required to engender health while bad air leads to disease: 'Air is as stagnant, musty, and corrupt as it can by possibly be made. It is quite ripe to breed small-pox, scarlet-fever, diphtheria, or anything else you please.' The notes start with the conviction that,

the very first canon of nursing, is the first and the last thing upon which a nurse's attention must be fixed, the first essential to a patient, without which all the rest you can do for him is as nothing, with which I had almost

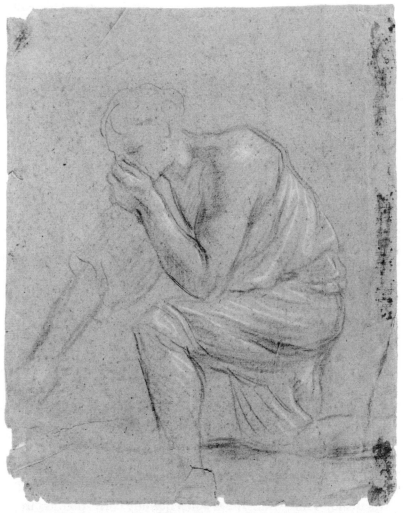

Drawing of a man holding his nose to avoid breathing in a miasma,
c. 17th century.

said you may leave all the rest alone, is this: TO KEEP THE
AIR HE BREATHES AS PURE AS THE EXTERNAL AIR, WITHOUT
CHILLING HIM.

Pure air was supplied through room ventilation by keeping
the windows wide open as much as possible when pure air was
believed to be available, such as at night when the patient slept
and factories were closed. 'The absence of smoke, the quiet, all

tend to make night the best time for airing the patients. One of our highest medical authorities on Consumption and Climate has told me that the air in London is never so good as after ten o'clock at night.'

Her view on bad air extends beyond the hospital ward, and she expounds her views on public health:

> I must say a word about servants' bed-rooms. From the way they are built, but oftener from the way they are kept . . . they are almost invariably dens of foul air, and the 'servants' health' suffers in an 'unaccountable' way, even in the country. For I am by no means speaking only of London houses, where too often servants are put to live under the ground and over the roof. [In] a country mansion . . . I have known three maids who slept in the same room ill of scarlet fever. 'How catching it is,' was of course the remark. One look at the room, one smell of the room, was quite enough.

Not only did the medical profession advocate fresh air but scientists and politicians as well, such as Benjamin Franklin. Jonathan Shipley, Bishop of St Asaph (1769–88), was a friend of Benjamin Franklin, and a colonial sympathizer during the American War of Independence. While living in Winchester, Franklin stayed with the bishop and became a family friend. The bishop's three daughters subsequently corresponded frequently with Franklin. In 1786 the second eldest of the daughters, Catherine, received a long letter from Franklin, who was then in Philadelphia, with the title 'The Art of Procuring Pleasant Dreams'. The letter begins with advice on the importance of eating well, good digestion and exercise. The latter part of the missive talks about what is needed to ensure good health: 'having a constant supply of fresh Air in your Bed chamber'. Franklin then describes how the air in an ill-ventilated room is tainted or spoiled. He refutes the idea held by physicians that fresh air is bad for you, and says that we should all sleep out in the open, or at least always with open bedroom windows, and 'put down the Glass of a coach' when travelling. He used the word 'aerophobic' to describe those who didn't advocate fresh ventilation. (Nowadays an aerophobic person is someone who is afraid of flying, a concept that did not exist in Franklin's time.) He concludes his letter with the advice that in order to get a good night's sleep, one needs 'what is necessary above all Things, a good Conscience'.

The miasma theory of disease finally lost favour following the work of the English physician and anaesthetist John Snow, who first expressed his ideas in his essay 'On the Mode of Communication of Cholera' (1849), followed by a treatise in 1855 convincingly showing that it was poor water quality rather than bad air that was the cause of cholera epidemics, such as the one in London between 1853 and 1854. This was the beginning of germ theory, which with the development of microscopy allowed specific organisms or germs to be identified as the cause of respiratory disease.

Expired air was known as viated air, and was thought to contain toxic substances, 'potamins the products of putrefactive decomposition'.[4] Oxygen was taken from the lungs and carbonaceous toxins returned in the darker, venous blood. Post-mortem evidence of this black carbonaceous waste was found in the lungs of deceased miners. Anoxia or lack of oxygen was not considered a problem. It was at the end of the nineteenth century that the vitiated air was carefully investigated using scientific techniques commonly used today. The person who did the most to transform people's fears and prejudices of vitiated air was the physiologist Haldane, who, by experimenting on himself and animals, showed that it was CO_2 that increases the breathing rate, not some unknown organic compounds.

Thomas H. Huxley, the Victorian biologist and well-known advocate of Charles Darwin and evolution, continued to believe that viated or expired air was obnoxious not because of the extra carbon dioxide it contained but because of unknown yet unidentified compounds. In his medical textbook of 1866, *Lessons in Elementary Physiology*, he states: 'Expired air contains in addition, small quantities of "animal matter" or organic impurities of a highly decomposable kind.' Despite these views and an intensive investigation, nobody could identify what these 'matters' were, but they were still thought to cause disease and illness. The Victorian public knew nothing of disease-causing agents such as bacteria, fungi and viruses. Huxley continued, 'Nothing is known of their nature, but they are probably the chief cause, why air which has been breathed once is extremely unwholesome if breathed a second time.'

The term 'malaria' is derived from an Italian colloquial word *mal' aria*, literally 'bad air' (from *mala*, bad, and *aria*, air), and was probably first used by the Italian physician Francisco Torti in the early eighteenth century. This term was introduced to the UK in 1827 by John MacCulloch.[5] Before this it had many names, such as marsh miasma, marsh fever and ague. Malaria manifests itself as a series of periodic fevers called tertian and quartan fevers.

Malaria is an ancient disease that has followed humankind throughout history and still causes around half a million deaths a year. It is a serious health hazard in parts of Africa and Asia, where babies and young children are the most vulnerable. Malaria is a complicated disease that results from infection with tiny blood-borne parasites of the genus *Plasmodium*. There are around four *Plasmodium* species that cause human malaria. The parasites sit in the salivary glands of female mosquitoes and are injected into the body when they pierce the skin and feed on blood. Female mosquitoes only need blood to lay eggs; otherwise, like the males, they are herbivores. Fortunately, only a few mosquito species transfer the parasites. They are from the *Anopheles* genus: while most of the other four hundred species are harmless, thirty mosquito species can carry *Plasmodium*. The parasite has a complex life cycle, going through many life stages, first in the mosquito and then in humans. Mosquitoes lay their eggs in still, warm and often stagnant water. In most cases, this is in swamps, pools and puddles. The association between malaria and living next to marshes provided the notion that malaria was caused by bad air that emanated from marshes and stagnant water and contained noxious vapours.

The discovery of malaria's cause was made in three stages: in the 1880s the human blood-borne parasites were discovered by the French army surgeon Charles Louis Alphonse Laveran, who received the 1907 Nobel Prize in Physiology or Medicine for his discovery. The life cycle of the parasite in the mosquito and the transmission of the parasite to humans from mosquitoes was described by Major Ronald Ross in India, where he was studying bird malaria.[6] He received the Nobel Prize in Physiology or Medicine in 1902 for these remarkable discoveries, becoming the first British Nobel laureate, and the first born outside Europe. Thus a fever thought to be caused by breathing a noxious miasma emitted from the ground turned out to be far more complicated than could be imagined.

Breathing, Influenza, Coronavirus and Airborne Disease

The Bible does not just express the spiritual role of breathing but offers medical observations as well. In the case of leprosy, for example, it provides the following advice in Leviticus 13:45: 'And the leper . . . shall cover his upper lip, and shall cry, "Unclean, unclean."' This implies that leprosy was thought to be passed on through the breath. It has only been established recently that infection with the leprosy bacteria, *Mycobacterium leprae*, occurs through breathing or nasal fluid, giving this biblical public-spirited advice relevance.[7]

Most people are unaware that leprosy can be transmitted via this route. The airborne disease we are most familiar with catching is a cold. The common cold is spread by a virus, rhinoviruses being the most common culprit. Rhinoviruses infect the upper respiratory tract, nose and throat, and cause a blocked, runny nose, a sore throat and a headache, making breathing laboured. Often the blocked nose leads to sneezing and coughing, which serves to clear your blocked airways but also gift the virus with a mechanism for being expelled widely into the air to be breathed in by the nearest person, and start the infection process all over again. When the virus infects the lower respiratory tract, the

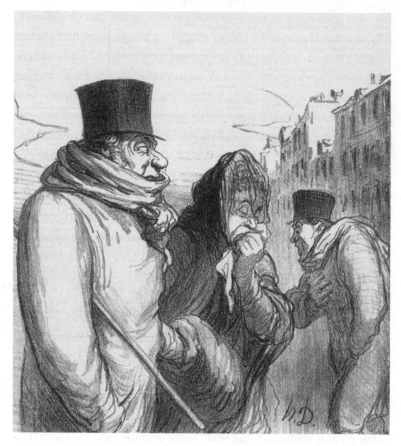

The Paris influenza 'Paris grippe' epidemic of 1864 depicted by Honoré Daumier, illustration from *Le Charivari*, 18 February 1864.

lungs, the cold becomes a lot more serious and is accompanied by plentiful coughing and mucus production. By adulthood virtually every human being in the northern hemisphere will have suffered a cold. When the symptoms are at their worst, people often think they must have the flu or influenza. Infection by the influenza virus alters your breathing in the same way as the rhinoviruses, but can be more severe, so severe that it can be fatal if caught by vulnerable people such as the elderly, pregnant women and children. Indeed, if a particularly infectious respiratory virus appears then global pandemics can occur, such as the recent Covid-19 pandemic, in which the minimization of the virus's transmission was attempted by the practice of physical distancing, ensuring a

2-metre (6½ ft) gap between people, and, more effectively, staying indoors as much as possible and avoiding social gatherings.

The pandemic with the highest mortality remains the 1918 influenza pandemic, which started during the First World War on the Western Front and ended on the home front after the war ended. It is believed that the first fatality, or the index patient, sometimes referred to as 'patient zero', was one Private Harry Underdown, who died at Hospital No. 24 in February 2017. His grave can be found in Étaples military cemetery in Pas-de-Calais, northern France. At Étaples, after Harry, a further 156 soldiers died in the following weeks. Why the flu started here can only be speculated, but Étaples was a coastal troop base combined with a supply depot, as it had good rail links. Thousands of horses were stabled there, which created mountains of manure. Added to this manure mountain were many piggeries and contributions from fowl such as ducks, geese and chickens. These farm animals were cared for by a large contingency of Chinese labourers recruited for the purpose by the British army. It was probably under these unhygienic, manure-ridden, tightly packed living conditions that the 'bird flu' virus jumped species to infect man and go on to ultimately kill more people in a few months than had been killed in combat during the whole of the war. In wintertime the atmosphere in the camp would have been damp, and inside it would have been full of dust, animal dander, bacteria, fungal spores and viruses, so it is no wonder that breathing this air would have allowed any respiratory infections to spread quickly.

Influenza epidemics are named after the geographical place where the index case was recorded. The 1918 pandemic is not known as French flu but Spanish flu, and later became called the Spanish Lady. During the closing stages of the war, the British, American and French presses were heavily censored, so negative news was not reported. The flu's devastating effect on both the health and mortality of the Allied soldiers never reached public notice. While the influenza was just as devastating to the Germans, this could not be reported either: some in the British military even thought it was a German plot. Eventually, as the flu spread across

Europe and the world, it reached Spain and Portugal, where it killed around 10 per cent of those infected. One notable victim was the Spanish king, Alfonso XIII, who was fortunate enough to recover. Spain, being neutral and not part of the war, allowed the Allied press to report the threat posed by this new strain of flu, thus giving it the name Spanish flu.[8]

This flu spread around the world, infecting around 500 million people and eventually killing an estimated total of 50 million. The death rate at its peak amounted to 60,000 a day. Nowadays a similarly virulent pandemic would result in a death toll amounting to hundreds of millions. We are better prepared, and every year the population is offered influenza vaccinations, which are tailored to defend against the most likely strains of the virus.

When influenza appeared, then as now, it struck overnight and after two to three weeks would subside. The 1918 influenza was unusual in that it infected the young and healthy, not the old and infirm. It overstimulated the body's immune response to the infection, and when pneumonia developed as a complication, it was often severe enough to kill.

Thus, in areas where overcrowding occurred, such as at military bases, transport ships and cinemas, it was particularly insidious. In some American cities the death rate rose sixfold with the flu and completely overwhelmed the public infrastructure, with nowhere to store the bodies and not enough coffins or even medical staff to treat the sick. In the UK the city of Nottingham was severely affected. The death rate of the 'ferocious epidemic' was so high that the Victoria Swimming Baths had to be drained to be used as a temporary morgue. In the end, the city recorded 60,000 flu deaths, the highest number in the UK.[9]

For most the flu would start with a headache and a raised temperature, but for those who suffered the most the symptoms were awful. They became cyanosed, exhibiting a blue tinge to their faces and lips that resulted from air hunger, their lungs slowly filling with pus. Difficulty in breathing was accompanied by copious nosebleeds and bloody airways. Flu sufferers were described generally as 'Blue as huckleberries and spitting blood'. There was nothing anyone could do, except lie in bed. If you survived the symptoms then after a few days the fever would pass, and you would soon feel better and return to normal. Many remedies were reported to be successful; sales of Vicks VapoRub and alcoholic drinks such as whisky skyrocketed. Drinking oxo cubes dissolved in hot water was another remedy recommended by many health professionals.

Viruses had yet to be discovered, so all infectious diseases were thought to be caused by bacteria. The medical profession argued as to the cause. Some thought it was a bacterium called Pfeiffer's bacillus, or *Bacillus influenzae*, which had first been isolated from infected nasal mucus in 1892 by Richard Pfeiffer, a leading German bacteriologist. The problem was that not everyone could find the bacteria, and when they did it was associated with other bacterial infections such as pneumonia, a secondary complication. The influenza virus was first isolated in 1933 in ferrets. These animals, along with guinea pigs, react to the virus infection in the same way as humans.[10] By the early 1940s the virus was incubated and grown in fertilized chicken eggs, allowing the production of the first primitive vaccines.[11]

There were many survivors of both the war and the flu. Some of these young survivors later became famous, such as Walt Disney, John Steinbeck, President Franklin D. Roosevelt and British prime minister David Lloyd George. Survival was a lottery. Joseph Burgess Wilson returned from the war to find his wife and daughter had both succumbed to the flu, the only survivor being his son. This son grew up to become the novelist Anthony Burgess, the author of *A Clockwork Orange*, who wrote of the event:

> My mother and sister dead. The Spanish Influenza pandemic had struck Harpurhey. There was no doubt of the existence of a God; only the Supreme Being could contrive so brilliant an afterpiece to four years of unprecedented suffering and devastation. I apparently was chuckling in my cot while my mother and sister lay dead on a bed in the same room.[12]

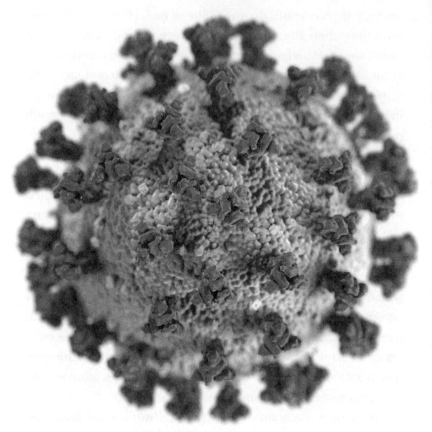

SARS-CoV-2 was the cause of the 2020 Covid-19 pandemic. The spikes adorning the surface give this group of viruses their coronal (or crown) nomenclature.

Since the Spanish flu there have been three major influenza pandemics: the Asian flu (1957–8), caused by the influenza virus A(H2N2), and the Hong Kong flu (1968–9), caused by the A(H3N2) virus. Each is estimated to have caused between 1 and 4 million deaths. Both pandemics were thought to be transferred from birds, particularly chickens, in regions where people live in close proximity to their birds. In 2009–10 a H1N1 virus appeared, but because of vaccination, only around 100,000 to 400,000 deaths were recorded, with children and the elderly being the most vulnerable.

The recent coronavirus pandemic is still fresh in everyone's mind, as the globe paused for most of 2020 and focused on halting the spread of the virus (named SARS-CoV-2, one of six human coronaviruses). Over many months, beginning in November 2019 in Wuhan, Hubei Province, China, it took just a matter of weeks to spread to virtually every country and community in the world, mainly by air travel, eventually infecting and killing millions. Only the remote island countries of the Pacific such as Vanuatu remained untouched. Once established in all the major cities of the world, infection rates took off steeply, with Europe and the USA recording the greatest infection and death rates. Unlike the 1918 influenza pandemic, this virus affected the elderly more than the young and healthy. This time older males with underlining health problems such as heart disease were the most vulnerable, followed by the elderly living together in social care and nursing homes. Many healthcare workers were infected by the virus, as they were unable to prevent it from entering their lungs through lack of effective breathing filtration of the ward air. Unfortunately many who received excessive virus exposure died, reflecting the fate of many of the nurses and doctors treating patients in the 1918 pandemic, just over one hundred years earlier.

The incubation time between exposure and exhibition of symptoms varied and averaged around five to six days. After this, the person was liable to spread the virus to others. Quarantine of around two weeks was needed for the infection to pass. Without quarantine, the new virus was easily spread in the air or by contact, typically infecting two or three other people, which caused an exponential explosion in cases. This began in China, and spread to the rest of the inhabited world. To slow this exponential rise, community 'lockdowns' and curfews became compulsory across most of the world. Isolation of families prevented person-to-person spread. Without this, the infection rate would have exploded, as it did with Spanish flu. This had huge implications for the world's economy: the majority of industry ceased as everyone stayed at home.

In the coronavirus pandemic, infection caused the condition known as Covid-19. Many people with Covid-19 exhibited such mild symptoms that the infection passed unnoticed. In those who did react to the virus, the principal symptoms were a persistent dry cough, a raised body temperature, manifesting as a slight fever, and body aches. Very rarely was there a runny nose or breathlessness. The symptoms lasted a few days and were followed by expectoration of mucus, with the temperature eventually subsiding to normal, the symptoms treatable with mild analgesics. More vulnerable people developed secondary symptoms, where the virus severely disrupted the airways, interfering with oxygen exchange. Breathing at this point becomes difficult and laboured. Here the body's immune response to the viral infection made people feel particularly ill and at their most vulnerable, especially when infected people were encouraged to self-isolate. In the majority of people, the infection cleared within a week or two of the appearance of the first symptoms. In those where the symptoms were more severe, hospitalization and close care was required with ventilatory support, receiving extra oxygen supplementation via a mask along with extra hydration.

In a small proportion of these patients, around 15 per cent, severe pneumonia developed, where the airways in the lungs fill with liquid, making breathing very difficult. A further 5 per cent developed acute respiratory distress syndrome (ARDS), septic shock and/or multiple organ failure and death.

In the 1918 influenza pandemic this pneumonia was a secondary bacterial infection, and people died quickly of hypoxia, but in the 2020 Covid-19 pandemic the pneumonia was new and different and resulted from the virus triggering an autoimmune response in which the body overacted to the infection. This difference suggested that treatment with anti-inflammatory drugs was worthwhile. Early in the epidemic physicians learnt that the simplest way to support the patient through these so-called 'cytokine storms' was to anaesthetize and fully sedate the person and support their breathing with mechanical ventilators, with each breath supplied via an endotracheal tube. This aspect of the epidemic had not been anticipated, so as the epidemic developed, an acute shortage of ventilators was predicted. Before the epidemic there were only a few thousand in use throughout the whole of the UK.

During the epidemic's first peak, thousands were required in London alone. Many died through lack of ventilators. The prime minister, Boris Johnson, famously asked U.S. President Donald Trump for extra ventilators. A few days later Johnson became infected with the virus and spent ten days in self-isolation before entering the second phase, where his breathing became difficult. He was supported in the intensive care unit of a hospital for three or four days using an oxygen mask. Constantly supervised by medical staff, he was never prescribed mechanical ventilation.

The majority of the first patients in China who succumbed to this virus worked or lived around a wholesale seafood market where live animals were also on sale. On sale as food, these animals are often kept in unhygienic conditions, providing an ideal environment for spreading viruses.

When and where the next airborne virus originates, whether it is via an animal vector or not, is unknown, but the next time a pandemic arises, we should hopefully find ourselves better prepared to combat its spread. We have yet to see how this new respiratory infection interacts with other respiratory infections, such as influenza and tuberculosis, and its impact on those tobacco smokers who suffer from COPD.

Modern Miasmas and Breathing Poisonous Gas

Another aspect of modern living we take for granted or expect is the use of electric lighting. At the flick of a switch, we light our rooms, setting them awash with a bright white light. Of course, this has not always been the case, and before the invention of the electric light, the dark was illumined by flames: at first the incidental light from burning wood, and then through the lighted wicks of candles. While these flames themselves do not render breathing difficult, the smoke and soot generated does. Breathing sooty air in a confined space night after dark night can lead to chronic lung diseases such as COPD (chronic obstructive pulmonary disease), a mixture of bronchitis and emphysema. Today in some parts of Africa wood is still used in cooking. A wood-burning

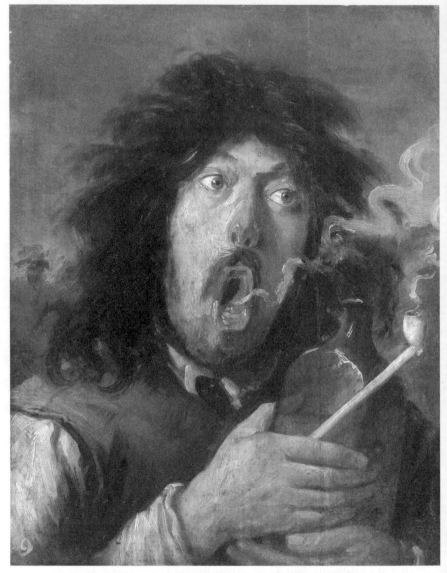

Joos van Craesbeeck, *The Smoker*, c. 1635–6, oil on panel.

fire requires close attention, so women (who do most of the cooking) often receive the greatest exposure to the smoke and develop COPD.

In eighteenth-century Europe new flammable gases were being discovered and synthesized, leading to a revolution in domestic and public lighting. The first in this revolution was the discovery of the element hydrogen, symbol H, by the English chemist Henry Cavendish in 1766. One day, taking a glass vessel filled with a mixture of his unknown 'inflammable air' (air and hydrogen), he applied a spark to it using a new piece of equipment, an electric generator. While the generated sparks arced across the glass, nothing dramatic happened, except that a small amount of mist appeared on the inner glass surface. Cavendish, wondering what the misting was, after further investigation found it to be water. To us this is not at all remarkable, but at the time this was an amazing discovery as it led to the notion that two gases, hydrogen and oxygen, could form a liquid when combined. Even more exciting, one of the gases, hydrogen, was inflammable (like oxygen). This research led to the identification of simpler (oxygen-free) flammable organic gases made of carbon and hydrogen, such as methane (formula CH_4).

An even more flammable gas was acetylene (C_2H_2), discovered accidentally in 1836 by Humphry Davy's cousin Edmund Davy, a chemistry professor. Acetylene produced a bright white, smokeless flame when burned. This property led to the gas being used in streetlamps and lighthouses. It was generated by dripping water onto powdered calcium carbide (CaC_2). Acetylene, when burnt cleanly in fresh air, had no negligible effect on breathing and the respiratory system, but it was noted to produce a slight 'garlicky' smell as it burnt. Generating the gas by adding water to powder was impractical for popular use and did not replace candle lighting.

Around this time, another inflammable carbon-based gas mixture appeared, known as coal gas, and later town gas. It was discovered that when coal was heated without oxygen, a dirty mixture of inflammable gases evolved. This gas mixture was a by-product of coke production (coke is used in iron ore smelting) and could be generated on an industrial scale. Someone soon realized that it could be easily stored in large pressurized gasometers near to where it was needed, and then piped to wherever it was required. A domestic network of piping soon grew, popularizing its use in cities and industry. These huge gasometers

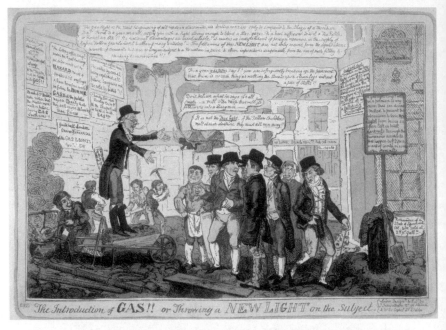

Satirical print, 'Introduction of gas!! Or throwing a new light
on the subject', 1815. An orator expounds to the public the benefits of piped
town gas in the London streets.

were a common feature of most town and city centres until quite
recently. Homes that received piped town gas used it at first to
light their homes, and then for cooking and heating. Initially
homes were lit with raw coal gas flames burning in wall-mounted
lanterns; these flames released tiny amounts of impurities into
the air, such as ammonia, sulphur and carbon monoxide, which
often made people ill and queasy. In addition the flames consumed the oxygen in the room, so sitting in a badly ventilated
room during the long dark winter evenings gave people headaches. More serious health problems could result if there was
a gas leak, including asphyxiation. The suppliers of coal gas of
course knew that it was toxic, as several suicides from breathing
coal gas (by placing one's head in an unlit oven, for example) were
reported, but decided to actively suppress this knowledge as they
did not want their sales to be hurt. Eventually the facts about town
gas toxicity leaked into the press, leading to town gas intoxica-
tion becoming a common method of suicide. Leaking odourless

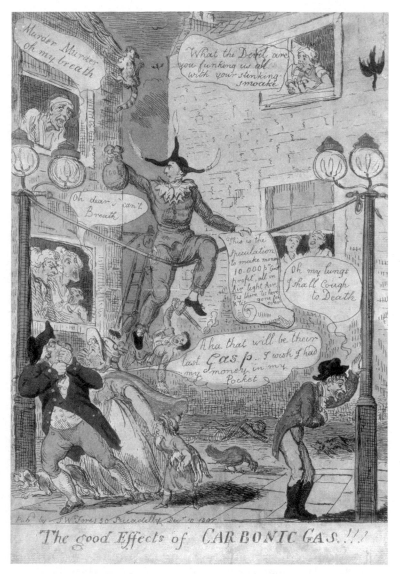

Isaac Cruikshank, 'Good effects of Carbonic Gas', 1807, hand etching.
A satirical print documenting the introduction of street lighting using lamps
that burned town gas, producing noxious fumes. The residents shown in
their night clothes are all complaining about the smell, and the acrobat
illustrates that money is being made by the suppliers.

gas could also cause explosions, so gas companies began to add tiny amounts of mercaptan, a sulphur-containing colourless gas that smells like rotten cabbage, even in very tiny amounts. Thus it was ensured that even the smallest gas leaks were detectable. Gradually town gas was replaced by natural gas, which is largely methane and burns more cleanly, producing water vapour and carbon dioxide. Natural gas permeates rocks deep beneath the Earth's surface and is obtained from wells. It is this carbon dioxide that is a major cause of climate change.

Any harm caused by breathing foul air in the home was unintentional. However, it was not long before chemists, the military and politicians realized that poison gas could be used to kill people on purpose.

Mass destruction by poisonous gas began in the First World War. Its first use as a weapon of mass destruction (WMD) was as an experiment by the German Army, near to the village of Langemarck, France, on 22 April 1915. It was late in the afternoon and the German, British and French forces had been shelling each other all day. The German experiment began when the wind was blowing in the right direction, away from the German trenches and towards the British and French trenches. Four divisions of the German 23rd and 26th Army Corps spaced along a 6.5-kilometre (4 mi.) front, when given the order, simultaneously unscrewed the release valves of 6,000 gas cylinders containing pressurized liquid chlorine. The released liquid quickly vaporized and soon formed a huge cloud of green chlorine gas. Chlorine gas is heavier than air, so in a light wind it will cling to the ground. The greenish-yellow cloud took around one minute to cross no man's land, where it soon engulfed thousands of unsuspecting Allied troops.

Unlike modern nerve agents, chorine is a simple poison. At high concentrations it destroys the lining of lungs. These then flood with a clear watery exudate, which when mixed with air foams up and blocks the airway. Asphyxiation results quickly, the person eventually drowning in their own bodily fluids.

Over the next hour it drifted another 16 kilometres (10 mi.) over enemy lines, becoming ever more dilute and at this point causing the troops mild irritation to their eyes and mouths. This single attack is estimated to have killed 5,000 troops and permanently injured another 10,000. For the Germans, the experiment was considered a great success and within an hour had punched a huge hole in the Allied defences. The Germans had not anticipated the spectacular effect of their experiment, however, so were not set to take advantage of the gap and move forward, therefore allowing the Allies to quickly repopulate the trenches once they realized the chlorine gas had dissipated.

Thirty-six hours later the Germans released a second chlorine gas cloud. Again the weather conditions were perfect, and, in this case, a light breeze carried the gas over the Canadian 8th Battalion. Thousands died in the trenches, as it was impossible to retreat from the gas cloud. Once one was engulfed, the act of running only increased the rate of breathing, and the more gas one breathed the quicker the chlorine damaged the lungs. Another 5,000 soldiers were killed, most within hours, but others took days, slowly dying, as their lung damage was irreparable. At first the Allies were taken by surprise and throughout May the Germans continued using chlorine in ever greater quantities, creating gas clouds with extremely toxic concentrations, which would remain lethal even after drifting for 16 kilometres or more. The Allied troops were quickly issued with crude respirators consisting of gauze soaked in soda lime. The soda itself would kill the soldiers if applied too liberally; some soldiers, thinking it was the gas that was killing them, would add more soda to the gauze, which would then asphyxiate them more. It did not take long for the British army to retaliate. On 25 September the British had accumulated 150 tonnes of chlorine gas on the Belgium front line at Loos.

During the First World War thousands of gas poisoning injuries were recorded, with 180,983 British alone, although the number of deaths was greatly under-reported at 6,062.[13] After the war, the chemical warfare that had occurred became an official state secret and all government documents on the subject remained classified for more than fifty years, with the facts not released until 1972.[14]

As the war progressed, research into noxious gas accelerated. The next gas to be used was phosgene, a molecular combination of chlorine, carbon and oxygen. It was originally named by its discoverer Humphry Davy, who in 1812 synthesized the chemical by exposing a mixture of carbon monoxide and chlorine to sunlight. *Phos* is derived from the Greek for 'light' and *gene,* born, so it means 'born from light'. Its name is the only good thing about the gas. Phosgene was used by both sides and caused even more death and casualties than chlorine. It proved more lethal, as when inhaled it was less irritating to the lungs and so produced less coughing, which allowed soldiers to inhale more deeply before they were aware of its presence. As a compound of chlorine, it still killed by asphyxiation, destroying the lining of the lungs, not always instantly but often days later. Killing and disabling its victims removed soldiers from the front line. Phosgene had its own peculiar smell, which at least gave some warning of its presence. Sometimes chlorine and phosgene were released at the same time.

In 1917 the Germans used a new agent on the Russian front line. This time chlorine and sulphur were combined to form a compound that smelled of mustard or garlic. Its chemical name was Bis (2-chloroethyl) sulphide, and it quickly became known as mustard gas. It was a fat-soluble oil as well, so as a gas it could enter the body through breathing, but as an oil it could enter the body through the skin. Another innovation was to deliver the compound in shells. Using artillery allowed it to be used precisely at a distance and along with ordnance shells. Mustard gas caused blistering internally and externally and prolonged death by many hours. A benefit but also a hindrance was that the oily compound could remain in the soil. This contaminated advancing troops trying to take advantage of an assault. By the end of 1917 over a third of shells held some form of poison gas, and if the war had continued, this proportion would have probably reached 50 per cent. A few days before the war ended, on 14 October 1918, the last Allied offensive was underway. The British were shelling the Belgian village Warwick with mustard shells. The village was held by the 16th Bavarian Reserve Infantry. The shelling was intense, and the Germans suffered heavy casualties. Among them was a young soldier, Adolf Hitler, who was injured and blinded by the mustard gas.[15]

Towards the end of the war, as the respirators issued to the troops became increasingly sophisticated, the simple noxious gases became ineffective. This then led to an acceleration of the chemical weapons arms race, leading to the development of even more deadly chemicals, the so-called nerve agents. These, when breathed in minute quantities, kill by paralysing the respiratory muscles. Death from respiratory failure and asphyxiation occur in minutes rather than hours or days. This arms race continued through the Cold War when the Novichok nerve agent was developed by the USSR. Novichok is a powder which in minute quantities clogs up the workings of the respiratory muscles by inhibiting the function of an enzyme called acetylcholinesterase, which modulates muscle contraction and relaxation. The agent stops the heart and paralyses the respiratory muscles, like the diaphragm, eventually leading to death by suffocation as the lungs fill with secreted fluid. Bad air indeed.

In 2018 the Russians decided to use this nerve agent in an assassination attempt on two of its citizens, the former Russian military officer and double agent Sergei Skripal and his daughter Yulia. Skripal was an exile living in the town of Salisbury, UK, where his daughter was visiting. They had become exposed to the agent after it had been smeared on the front door handle of his house. On 3 March they went to Salisbury's town centre for a meal and were found two hours later foaming at the mouth and struggling for breath in a nearby park. A passing doctor and nurse had spotted them, and the victims were rushed separately to hospital, where they were given intensive respiratory support. Yulia was discharged from hospital in April and her father a month later. In June, Dawn Sturgess and Charlie Rowley were exposed to Novichok. They had found a discarded container in a local park in Amesbury (near Salisbury). The container was camouflaged as a perfume bottle, so Dawn sprayed herself with the 'oily' contents;

she became ill instantly and died eight days later. Rowley survived. (The Alexei Navalny case in August 2019 shows that this agent is still being used to poison people.)

Before the First World War the Hague Declaration of 1899 had been crafted to define the boundaries of what was then modern warfare: what was considered civilized behaviour and what was not. When it came to gas warfare the Germans, who were signatories, ignored the declaration that contained a pledge 'to abstain from the use of projectiles, the sole object of which is the diffusion of asphyxiating or deleterious gases'. The Germans denied breaking the terms, at first as no projectiles were used. To them, using poisonous gas alone was not uncivilized. The Germans felt they were forced to use these new weapons because the Allies, via a naval blockade, were preventing nitrate imports from reaching Germany, limiting the country's ability to make explosives. They had a well-developed chemical industry that was well equipped to make chlorine gas on an industrial scale. The Germans also knew that the Allies had no capacity to make industrial quantities of chlorine, so could not retaliate.

In the history of breathing we come across the German chemist Fritz Haber (1868–1934), the inventor of chemical warfare, who in 1923 stated: 'In no future war will the military be able to ignore poison gas. It is a higher form of killing.'[16] At the age of fifty he received the 1918 Nobel Prize in Chemistry for his brilliant work on the direct synthesis of ammonia (NH_3) from nitrogen (N_2) and hydrogen (H_2), completed in 1909. Plants can use ammonia as a source of nitrogen to produce proteins and DNA. Using the Haber process on an industrial scale allowed Germany and the rest of the world to synthesize unlimited supplies of cheap fertilizers. Haber sold the rights to his process and became wealthy. Being a German patriot, he joined the Ministry of War when the First World War began, where he worked on converting his process to make explosives and to synthesize petrol from coal. During this period he switched to gas warfare and weaponized chlorine gas, personally attending its first use at Ypres in 1915. After this release Haber became a great enthusiast of gas warfare. While on his way to the Russian front, he visited his home for a few days' break, to see his wife, Clara, who was also a chemist. Clara was so opposed to her husband's jingoistic views that on his first night home, while Haber slept, she took his service revolver and went into the garden, where she fatally shot herself in the head. The suicide was unfortunately witnessed by her young son, Hermann. Clara's suicide had a negligible effect upon Haber and he soon married again.

After the war he oversaw the development of a cyanide gas formulation, for the peaceful purpose of being used as an insecticide. The gas was called Zyklon A (Cyclone A), and it had already been used as a chemical weapon in the war. Haber died at the age of 65 in January 1934 while travelling through Switzerland on his way to Palestine, where he had been offered a directorship at the Sieff Research Institute (now the Weizmann Institute). Later, a new even more lethal formulation was made, Zyklon B, which was adopted by the Nazis in concentration camps such as Auschwitz and used to gas and kill millions of Jews. Haber, being Jewish, lost many of his relatives in this way. Later, his son Hermann moved to the USA, where he committed suicide in 1946, followed later in 1949 by his daughter Claire, Haber's granddaughter, who was working on an antidote to the effects of chlorine gas. She killed herself when she was told her work was no longer needed, as work on the atomic bomb was considered more important by the U.S. authorities.

Modern Miasma

Even today, unusual, mysterious miasma can appear without notice. This happened in Cameroon on 21 August 1986 when a natural disaster of biblical proportions occurred at Lake Nyos, a crater lake of volcanic origin in the Oku plain in northwest Cameroon.[17] In the night, while everyone slept, a huge gaseous miasma belched up from the bottom of the lake, ultimately killing 1,746 people, around 6,000 cattle and almost every living creature near the shoreline. It has been estimated that in that one event, around a quarter of a million tons (1.147 million cubic metres) of carbon dioxide was released into the air. Unbeknown to anyone, the carbon dioxide had been slowly building up on the lake floor over many months and years. The cataclysmic release of this miasmic mixture of water vapour and CO_2 rolled over the lake and down the surrounding mountainside to villages in the valley below. The sleeping villagers were exposed to nearly pure CO_2; anything above 30 per cent CO_2 is enough to render the breather unconscious. Thus thousands of villagers passed out and lay comatose in their beds. While thousands eventually recovered as the gas cloud drifted away, 1,746 did not. Today the lake is monitored, and deep water is purposely pumped to the surface where it is circulated with the surface water in the hope that CO_2 levels will never reach such dangerous levels again.

The Lake Nyos disaster death-toll was high as it occurred at night when people slept. While asleep we are less conscious of toxic gases and can soon succumb to asphyxiation. Thus, many domestic deaths from breathing noxious substances occur at night. Most of these deaths are associated with domestic gas

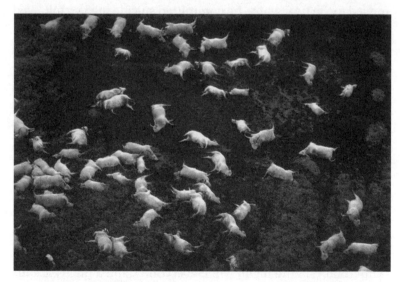

The Lake Nyos disaster of August 1986 in northwestern Cameroon.
A cloud of carbon dioxide was released from the lake and rolled down over the local villages, asphyxiating around 1,700 people alongside their livestock and the local fauna.

appliances, such as boilers, but this has not always been the case. A domestic technology that has played a role in this history is the refrigerator. To be effective refrigerators require liquid coolants that boil or turn to gaseous vapours at low temperatures. In the earliest commercial refrigerators of the 1920s these vapours were poisonous if inhaled. Coolants such as methyl chloride, sulphur dioxide or ammonia were used.[18] These liquids were pumped around the fridge under pressure, so if the piping leaked, which they often did, then lethal gases quickly filled the air. Inevitably several families were fatally poisoned in their homes by their fridges springing a leak while they slept. This led to scientists, even Albert Einstein, trying to design less fatal fridges, but with limited success. A more successful approach was to use coolants that weren't toxic when inhaled. This wasn't achieved until 1928, when an employee of General Motors, chemist Thomas Midgley Jr, together with his colleague Charles Franklin Kettering, synthesized freon. Freon is carbon-based, like oil, but instead of being bejewelled with hydrogen atoms, the carbon chain is decorated with fluorine and chlorine atoms. Freon is a liquid or gas that is colourless, odourless, non-flammable and non-corrosive. This was a major discovery and Midgley was lauded for it. He was so confident of its inert nature that he demonstrated the physical properties of his new coolant to the American Chemical Society by inhaling a lung full of it and then extinguishing a lighted candle by slowing exhaling the gas across the flame.

Not until the 1980s was it discovered that freon was not totally inert and when exposed to ultraviolet light in the stratosphere, the upper atmosphere, it reacts with the ozone (O_3) layer. This layer filters out excessive ultraviolet light, which can be damaging to most organisms when they are exposed to excessive amounts. The coolant freon and its chemical relatives had created a large ozone hole over Antarctica. Each year it seemed to be getting bigger and bigger. A total ban on freon use was agreed with the global ratification of the Montreal Protocol in 1987.

In 1921 Thomas Midgley developed what inadvertently turned out to be another poisonous substance, tetraethyl lead, which was added to petrol to allow it to burn more efficiently, increasing engine performance. Alcohol wasn't the only substance that does this: ethanol also will. This could not be patented, but tetraethyl lead could be, so once production was scaled up, the chemical made vast profits. Leaded petrol soon became universal until it was eventually banned in the early 2000s in Europe, having already been banned in the late 1990s in the U.S. and UK. The lead in children's blood had reached alarming levels, especially those exposed to car exhaust fumes from living near main roads. Lead is a respiratory toxicant and as a result of his research Thomas Midgley permanently damaged his lungs. In 1923 he wrote, 'I find that my lungs have been affected and that it is necessary to drop all work and get a large supply of fresh air.' He kept this disability a secret all his life, which wasn't all that long: he died in 1940 at the age of 51. Along with his respiratory problems, he contracted polio, which, combined with his damaged lungs, reduced his mobility considerably. To overcome this he invented a complicated system of pulleys and ropes which would allow him to raise himself from his bed each morning unassisted. Unfortunately, one morning it all went wrong, and he ended up entangling himself in the ropes and died of asphyxiation via strangulation.

The toxicity of lead has been known for hundreds of years, with long-term exposure damaging the nervous system and kidney function. Lead is a common, soft metal that is easy to work, so its toxicity has been overlooked; thus lead exposure has occurred through being added to petrol, being used in lead pipes carrying drinking water, ceramic glazes, soldering from canned foods, and traditional medicines.[19] Lead carbonate forms a snow-white pigment called lead white, which has been used as a pigment in paint around the world since ancient times (now replaced by the less toxic titanium dioxide). Its production required soaking sheets of lead in vinegar and exposing it to the air.[20] This was deadly for the paint makers. In 1677 Sir Philiberto Vernatti published an article, 'A Relation of the making of Ceruss,' in the *Philosophical Transactions of the Royal Society of London*: he stated that 'It brings them acute fevers, and great Asthma's or

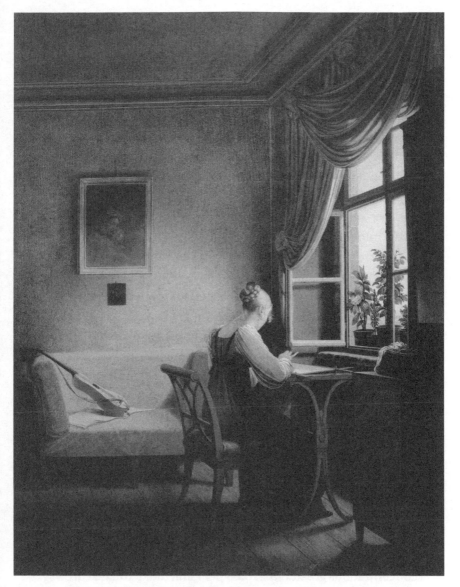

Georg Friedrich Kersting, *Embroidery Woman*, 1817, oil on panel. A domestic room decorated in Scheele's green.

shortness of breath.'[21] Since then many people have ruined their lungs through exposure to lead vapours.

Another dye that alters breathing is Scheele's green. Invented by the Swedish chemist Carl Wilhelm Scheele, who discovered oxygen, the compound copper arsenite presents as a vivid pea green colour. It soon became fashionable as a pigment and dye, particularly in wallpaper patterns, reaching its peak of popularity by the 1860s. Then, worrying reports about its toxicity began to appear in the press. People who had decorated their living rooms and bedrooms with this bright-green wallpaper complained of feeling ill and finding the rooms vaguely uncomfortable. Occupants became breathless after a few hours' occupation. The damp walls, and the flour-based wallpaper paste used to hang the paper, allowed a mould, *Scopulariopis brevicaulis*, to grow under the paper. This would then metabolize the arsenic to produce a garlicky-smelling toxic gas called trimethylarsine, which passes easily into the blood when breathed in.

After a campaign in the press, Scheele's green was abandoned. Its toxicity was soon forgotten, but it was remembered by Agatha Christie, the crime writer, who referred to it in her 1951 novel *They Came to Baghdad*. In the novel Sir Rupert Crofton Lee arrives at Baghdad aerodrome, where he is met by the young Mr Lionel Shrivenham of the British Embassy, much to the affront of Sir Rupert, who is expecting to be met by a more senior staff member. The Oriental Counsellor Mr Rice is ill with a 'Violent type of gastroenteritis. Something a bit worse than the usual Baghdad tummy.' Sir Rupert, being informed of this, frowns and asks 'if it might be a case of Scheele's Green', or arsenic poisoning.

Exposure to poisonous gases both natural and unnatural is common, but one of the most common and lethal is carbon monoxide, CO. The symptoms of carbon monoxide poisoning are insidious, creeping up slowly as each breath increases the quantity of gas absorbed into the blood. Toxic blood levels, at air concentrations greater than 0.08 per cent, make you feel drowsy. Often people exposed to CO are asphyxiated and look as if they are asleep at higher levels of concentration, around 1 per cent being lethal. CO and CO_2 have a similar chemical formula, so why is CO far more toxic than CO_2, as the only difference between the two molecules is a single oxygen atom? Inhaled CO quickly passes through the lungs into the blood, where it binds to the haemoglobin molecule in the red blood cells. CO binds more tightly to the haemoglobin molecule than oxygen, which displaces and prevents the oxygen binding, forming carboxyhaemoglobin instead of oxyhaemoglobin. Thus less oxygen gets to the tissues and cells die from asphyxiation. People with CO poisoning often have a healthy-looking pink tinge to their skin; this mimics the look of fully oxygenated blood, which we see when we blush.

History is littered with cases of carbon monoxide poisoning, which have occurred ever since humans sat around communal fires to cook, stay warm and socialize. Most of these smoky communal fires were lit in poorly ventilated spaces. The Roman emperor Julian the Apostate (331–363) nearly died from CO poisoning after having a burning coal-brazier placed in his apartment. Luckily, he was discovered, and his unconscious body was taken outside, where in the fresh air he made a full recovery. In more modern times accidental poisoning has often occurred in insufficiently ventilated spaces, especially in railway tunnels, when steam-driven locomotives produced copious amounts of smoke. One particular occasion was in 1944, when five hundred passengers were killed after a train stalled inside a tunnel in Balvano, Italy. During the Second World War, the Nazis realized the potential of CO and intentionally fatally poisoned around 700,000 people with it during the 1930s and '40s. Today deaths from CO poisoning continue as a result of poorly maintained gas boilers or cookers, or blocked flues. Blockages can lead to the CO concentration rising to lethal levels very quickly. In the USA, between 1999 and 2012, there were 6,136 CO-related deaths, around 438 annually, while the UK saw 148 in 2017.[22]

The production of carboxyhaemoglobin by CO is one way to cause hypoxia. Another is via the formation of methaemoglobin, which is created by nitrite ions (NO_2) binding to the haemoglobin and displacing the oxygen. The nitrite oxidizes the iron in haemoglobin to another form (called a trivalent state, 3^+), just like rusty iron, which gives the blood a brownish colour. This, when seen through the veins, gives the tissue a blue or lavender colour, different to the heliotrope or violet colour seen in normal deoxygenated blood. The first recorded deaths from methaemoglobinaemia occurred in 1945 when an American paediatrician, Hunter Comly from Iowa City, reported the deaths of two newborn babies from infantile methaemoglobinaemia in rural Iowa. The cause was unknown, and he called it 'blue baby syndrome'. He speculated on its cause and eventually decided that it was due to contaminated well water, positing that the well water used to make up the babies' formula contained too much nitrate, which is converted to nitrite once in the body.[23] A closer inspection of these farm wells showed that they were very unhygienic and not very well differentiated from the farm's sewage systems. In the USA, this study led in 1951 to a 48-state survey, and 278 'blue-baby' cases were identified, with 39 deaths; none were identified from before the Second World War or from babies who were breastfed.[24] This led to new worldwide guidelines on the upper limits of nitrate in drinking water. With these guidelines in use cases of infantile methaemoglobinaemia (the clinical name for blue baby syndrome) disappeared, until mysteriously, between 1983 and 1996, 93 new cases were reported; these were puzzling, as water nitrate seemed to have nothing to do with the epidemic. Since 1996, only two cases have been reported, and the condition has disappeared as quickly as it appeared. In 1999 the American environmentalist

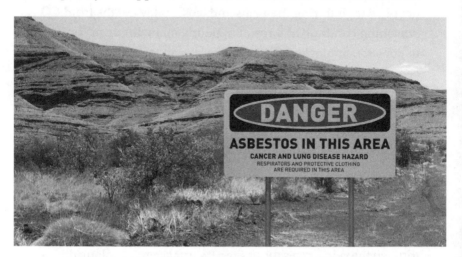

A warning sign from the asbestos-contaminated area of Wittenoom, Australia, in 2016, warning that respirators and protective clothing must be worn when entering the site.

Alex Avery speculated that this infantile methaemoglobinaemia was related to infant inflammatory bowel disease, where the gut bacteria converted the nitrate to nitrite.[25] If this is the cause, then we may not need to maintain a low water nitrate concentration.

Another mineral that was thought inert was asbestos, a fibrous silicate mineral that has been in use since Neolithic times as a building material and more recently as a non-flammable insulating material used to line pipes and line ceilings. Asbestos is fibrous, soft and easily crumbles to form a fine dust. These fine asbestos dust fibres, when breathed in, can reach deep inside the lungs and become permanently lodged in the lung lining. Prolonged exposure results in asbestosis (similar to pneumoconiosis) and lethal cancers such as lung cancer, and, particular to asbestosis, malignant mesothelioma. Breathing with mesothelioma is painful and debilitating. In 1937 in Wittenoom, Western Australia, mineral prospectors came across an abundant supply of crocidolite (blue asbestos).[26] World commodity prices were sufficiently high to make mining profitable. This started with digging the asbestos exposed on the surface and then transporting it 320 kilometres (200 mi.) by donkey to the nearest port. With the Second World War, demand for asbestos rose quickly, allowing the Australian Blue Asbestos Ltd to expand their mining activity considerably to meet the demand, eventually reaching a peak production of 17,490 tons in 1962. Due to the remoteness of the deposit, most of the miners lived nearby with their families in the town of Wittenoom, which had a population of 20,000, a police station, hotel and shops. In the 1950s the first cases of asbestosis in the miners were noted. By 2013, 143 miners and 10 residents had died from it, even though the mine had been closed since 1966. The first cases of mesothelioma appeared a little later in the 1960s, along with the first cases of lung cancer. By 2015 the mortality rate was 3,822 workers and 1,443 residents. The high death rate among the residents was due to the fact that asbestos dust blanketed the village, with few attempting to prevent it or clean it up. Children played freely in back gardens and went swimming at Wittenoom gorge, despite everywhere being coated with asbestos fibres.

Wittenoom is now a ghost town, its structures demolished and roads removed, with most of its residents were relocated to Perth. A few people stayed even after the town was officially removed from the map. It was too expensive to clear the asbestos and visitors today are warned not to enter the area without ventilator masks. This industrial disaster continues, as many of the residents were children when they left and will have to wait and see how their health develops, despite the fact that they are now breathing clean fresh air.

Breathing toxic air still happens, as in the steel town of Corby in Northamptonshire in the UK. In 1985 dust from a reclamation site containing cadmium, which is toxic and can enter the blood via the lungs, was breathed in by several pregnant women living nearby, who subsequently gave birth to children with limb reduction defects, such as hands with fingers missing. This was the first recorded case in the world in which unborn children were affected by air pollution.

Ventilation and Fresh Air

In the Victorian period, with the Industrial Revolution in full-swing, access to fresh air to breathe became limited, as smoke, poor sanitation and putrification went uncontrolled. In towns and cities, the air was polluted and smelly. Thus the concept of hygienic ventilation was born. This idea was soon reflected in construction advice, as construction was occurring on a vast scale. Cities grew at an unprecedented rate as people moved from the countryside to work in factories in towns and cities. Creating a healthy house with hygienic ventilation required the builder to consider its surrounding climatological and geological conditions.[27] This included a check on the soil surrounding the house, as well as the thickness of the walls. Wall thickness dictated how well the air would ventilate through the windows and thus contribute to the health of the occupants. Recommendations stated that the soil should be well drained and a damp course added to the walls, but above all, the external walls had to be exposed 'to aerial currents'

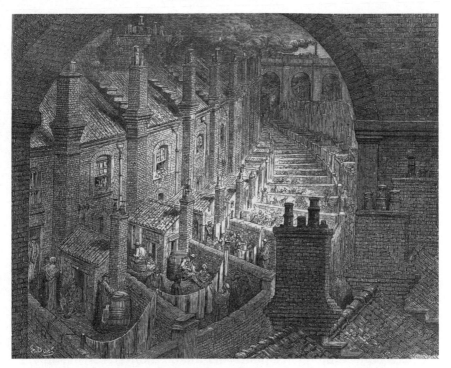

Gustave Doré, 'Over London-by Rail', 1872, wood engraving. With rapid Victorian urbanization and high occupancy rates, little consideration was given in the British capital to environmental conditions or public health.

and 'be permeable' enough to allow agreeable ventilation. These considerations were fine for suburban and rural dwellers, but not for the urban dwellers of the big cities, such as London and Manchester, where houses were squeezed tightly together in rows and terraces and little regard was given to ventilation or open space. These houses were often occupied by large extended families. A contemporary text states that they had little room for ventilation: 'Insufficient oxygenation caused much chloro-anaemia and many other maladies which rage with such intensity in populous centres.'[28]

Not all was doom and gloom, and some cities, such as Paris, had regulations regarding overcrowding. Here the breadth of the street had to match the height of the house, or vice versa. Attempts were made in the UK to do likewise. There, receiving enough light was considered more important than space. To receive sufficient sunlight, it was suggested that rooms occupied in the daytime should face southeast, while bedrooms should face east, and the least occupied rooms, such as the dining room, kitchen and closets, north.

When it came to healthy breathing, room size was considered the most important factor. It was estimated that 1,000 cubic feet (28 m³) of space was required per room occupant, a space of 10 by 10 by 10 feet (3 × 3 × 3 metres), with this space receiving 3,000 cubic feet (85 m³) of fresh air per hour. These generous spaces can be found in the Edwardian and Victorian houses of the wealthier classes, but not in the homes of the less fortunate. These ventilation figures were based on the notion that exhaled air contained noxious unidentified substances or 'bad air'. These unidentified substances turned out to be carbon dioxide, carbon monoxide and coal smoke. The ideal ventilation rate was calculated accordingly. Starting with the assumption that each person or room occupant produced 0.6 cubic feet (17 l) of CO_2 per hour, this would raise the CO_2 concentration in a poorly ventilated room (receiving only 1,000 cubic feet per hour) to 0.1 per cent (from 0.03 per cent in fresh air) in a few hours. Only by ventilating with 3,000 cubic feet of air per hour could the room concentration of CO_2 fall to an acceptable 0.06 per cent. While today there are minimum recommended internal CO_2 levels, they are much higher than 0.1 per cent. The excessive Victorian and Edwardian ventilation rates are more likely those needed to facilitate the dilution and expulsion of smells from body odour, as bathing and frequent washing of clothes was not as common as it is today.

Even today, we ventilate many of our rooms, particularly bathrooms, kitchens and bedrooms, heating them with fan heaters in the winter, cooling them with air conditioners in the summer and using extractor fans all year round to remove unwanted odours. Overall, we provide air that is pleasant to breathe. To enhance this sensation, we buy fragrant air sprays and solvents to release scent into our homes. The most popular smells are plant-based botanicals. Oddly, we even burn candles for this purpose, which produce pleasurable scents but invisible smoke and soot. We add further floral scents to our washing machines, and fragrance ourselves with deodorants, soaps and perfumes.

This notion that poor ventilation and viated air contributed to ill health and contagious disease was popular with the press. An article from the *Pictorial Times* in April 1846 warned churchgoers of the dangers of prolonged church services.

No buildings are more deficient in ventilation than places of public worship. Air loaded with the products from the consumption of gas, oil and candles, chilling draughts from an immense surface of glass, inequality of heat, emanations from graveyards and sometimes from dead bodies under pews in the very centre of the building, and in some places the poisonous emanations of an open charcoal brazier passing from the corridor into the church, may all be observed producing a deleterious effects.

A connection with death was also well-publicized, as illustrated by an 1812 epitaph for three well-diggers in a Yorkshire church graveyard.[29] The three unfortunates died while

venturing into a well at Marton when it was filled with carbonic acid gas, or fixed air. From this unhappy accident let others take warning not to venture into wells without first trying whether a candle will burn to the bottom, they may be entered with safety. If it goes out human life cannot be sustained.

In big cities such as London and Paris, one consequence of the increasing population density was that burial grounds became full. Soon a number of church graveyards only had room to expand downwards. Deeper and deeper graves were dug, the largest with a capacity of around eighteen coffins, vertically stacked in pairs on top of one another. While these graves were being filled, it was customary practice to leave them open, which often left the residents living next to graveyards complaining of the putrid smell, particularly during hot weather. A freshly decomposing body emits many gases: simple gases, such as carbon dioxide, methane and hydrogen sulphide, and other more complex organic ones that smell unpleasant, such as putrescine (1,4-diaminobutane), which nowadays is actually produced synthetically to make nylon. Despite its name, putrescine is made naturally by our cells but only in small quantities, and when noticed contributes to the smell of bad breath. Another unpleasant-smelling organic compound is cadaverine. These compounds can be toxic at raised concentrations and gravediggers would have to ensure that their partially filled graves were safe and adequately ventilated before entering. This was not always the case and fatal accidents happened. One such occasion was in September 1838, when Thomas Oakes died while at the bottom of a partially filled grave pit, which was over 17 metres (55 ft) in depth. To make matters worse, his first rescuer, young Edward Luddett, died instantly as he entered the pit as well. The two dead men were eventually withdrawn from the grave using a rope and meat hook supplied by the local butcher.

The two deaths and the subsequent inquest were reported in the national press and led to changes in the way bodies were

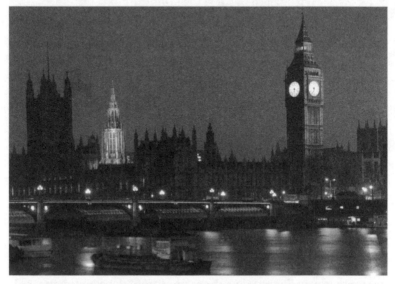

Houses of Parliament, London, from the South Bank, with the central ventilation tower illuminated.

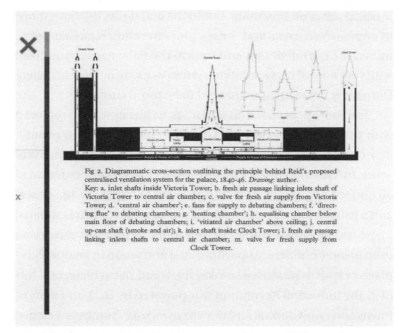

Fig 2. Diagrammatic cross-section outlining the principle behind Reid's proposed centralised ventilation system for the palace, 1840-46. *Drawing*: author.
Key: a. inlet shafts inside Victoria Tower; b. fresh air passage linking inlets shaft of Victoria Tower to central air chamber; c. valve for fresh air supply from Victoria Tower; d. 'central air chamber'; e. fans for supply to debating chambers; f. 'directing flue' to debating chambers; g. 'heating chamber'; h. equalising chamber below main floor of debating chambers; i. 'vitiated air chamber' above ceiling; j. central up-cast shaft (smoke and air); k. inlet shaft inside Clock Tower; l. fresh air passage linking inlets shafts to central air chamber; m. valve for fresh supply from Clock Tower.

Illustration (1840-46) of the historic ventilation system of the House of Commons, 1840-52, illustrating how air is drawn from both ends of the palace, from Victoria tower to Elizabeth tower (Big Ben) and expelled through the central tower.

buried. Deep graves were outlawed. By the 1860s most of the London cemeteries were closed. Bodies were removed and re-interred in new garden cemeteries outside the city, such as in Highgate. In Paris a different solution has been found: from the 1780s remains were removed to catacombs under the city streets.[30]

Once ventilation was taken seriously, all new buildings were purposefully designed to provide every occupant with a fresh supply of air to facilitate breathing, and to naturally ventilate away stale expired breath. When the new Palace of Westminster was built between 1840 and 1876, the Scottish physician David Boswell Reid designed an extensive ventilation system in the 1840s with this in mind. His design provided a flow of fresh air through the debating chambers, allowing fresh air to be drawn up from vents near the floor. The viated air would be extracted through vents in the ceiling and pulled up into towers where the air would be exhausted to the atmosphere. The design was based on Reid's medical views on breathing, but in the end it was the limitations of architecture, costs and the incumbent politicians that determined the overall design and in 1876 the Palace was completed with very little of his ventilation system working or even installed. Ultimately the ventilation proved to be too 'draughty'.[31]

The concept of viated air and miasma has now been replaced with the term 'air pollution'. Air pollution seems like a twenty-first-century phenomenon but has been around for hundreds of years. In Victorian times fireplaces and chimneys were found in all houses. A fireplace and chimney with or without a fire generates a considerable flow of fresh air through the room it is situated in, providing good ventilation, but in the winter this creates an even greater problem, as burning coal and wood in an open fireplace or hearth produces smoke, thick and particulate, and lots of it. The Industrial Revolution was powered by coal, and in most towns and cities dozens and dozens of factory chimneys belched out smoke all day, while domestic fires in the surrounding back-to-back houses did so day and night. On windy days the smoke was blown away, and the city dwellers received clear air. But, on occasions when the outside air was still and cold, fog would form, which then often mixed with the smoke and created a thick mixture we call smog. The same also happened when a warm layer of air sitting over a town or city trapped the colder air underneath, a so-called 'temperature inversion'. In Victorian London, where cheap and poor-quality coal with a high sulphur content was burnt, any smog that formed contained not only soot (carbon) but sulphur dioxide, imparting a greenish or yellow tinge to the smog. This thick greenish smog attracted the sobriquet of 'pea-souper'. Not only did the smog make the air smell sulphurous but it left a metallic taste in the mouth and irritated the nose, throat and eyes, making them water as they do when you peel onions. It even made smoking unpleasant. Those with chronic respiratory disease found it even harder to breathe and sometimes those affected with particular severe symptoms suffered early death.

These frequent smogs spurred the public into action, and many new Smoke Abatement societies were formed across most of the industrialized cities and towns of the UK. These early environmental groups of activists campaigned for smoke-free air for everyone but were in the minority. The reason was that the working public were more worried about their employment than the occasional smog, as most of the big local employers were factory-based. In a typical sentiment of the time, 'The [worker] would be sorry to see a persecution commenced against the manufacturers, for if they were driven from the borough where would the bread of the working man come from.'[32]

The government was not interested in the problem; for them the responsibility of maintaining clean air belonged to local governments and councils. This made it difficult to control pollution, as smoke does not respect borders, and often the smoke came from somewhere outside of their jurisdiction. Finally, in 1914 a UK-wide approach was advocated. However, nothing happened with the arrival of industrialized warfare of the First World War.

The Big Smoke

Air pollution is not a new phenomenon. Owing to its geography and climate, London regularly experiences periods when it is covered in a blanket of still air. Under these conditions smoke sits in the air. This started in the thirteenth century, when coal burning began, and although it was worse by the 1600s it wasn't until the 1900s that it began to become unhealthy.[33] The smog reached its zenith in 1952. For four days and nights (Friday to Tuesday, 5–9 December) London was shrouded in a thick pea-green smog. Visibility was reduced to a few metres and made driving above walking speed impossible. Navigating the streets on foot was difficult as pedestrians could not see their feet and had to shuffle around in case they tripped over kerbs and the like. People found breathing difficult and some wore masks or breathed through handkerchiefs, all to no effect.

It was after the 1952 smog that London hospitals were overwhelmed with people with respiratory problems. An unprecedented number of around 150,000 people were hospitalized and

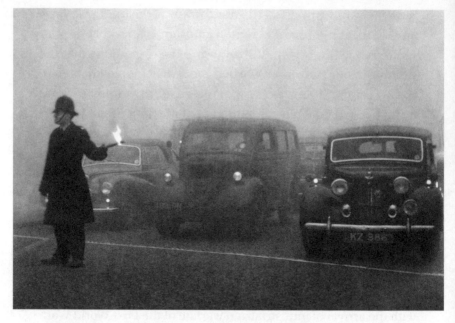

Policeman on traffic duty seen here using flares to guide the traffic during heavy smog in London, 8 December 1952.

around 12,000 lost their lives. This ill health was quickly associated with the toxicity of the mixture of gases in the 'pea-souper' smog. The appalling death rate spurred the government and parliament to finally act and in 1956, Queen Elizabeth II enacted the Clean Air Act. Anti-pollution legislation still had many detractors and the bill had to be pushed through by a select committee and supported by backbenchers; the Conservative government remained sceptical. The Clean Air Act meant that only smokeless coal could be used in populated areas.

The exact chemistry behind smog formation has only recently been worked out. Current smog studies show that sulphur introduced into the air forms a sulphate, which is catalysed by any nitrous oxide present. This, coupled with a high humidity, low temperature and large fog droplets, creates a thick smog.[34] It also leads to significant concentrations of sulphuric acid being generated in the fog/smog. Londoners exposed to the 1952 smog had their lungs burned by this acid. Nowadays the smogs experienced in the big Chinese and Indian cities are the same in composition, just far more expansive and more lethal, killing hundreds of thousands of people per year.

According to the World Health Organization, in 2019 air pollution caused the death of 7 million people every year. It accounts for a third of fatalities from strokes, lung cancer and heart disease, with more than 90 per cent of children breathing toxic air every day. Today in Europe it is not sulphur from coal-burning industries but nitrous oxide and small nano-sized carbon particles from traffic that is doing the damage. This pollution is expelled from the exhaust pipes of petrol- and diesel-powered vehicles: cars, vans, buses and lorries.

It is a great tragedy that even today most city-dwellers are breathing polluted air, and that young children are most at risk. The reason for this is one of political priorities and unforeseen consequences. In the 1990s, when it was realized that the lead from leaded petrol was particularly neurotoxic to children, production across the world ceased, and it was banned from petrol worldwide by the early 2000s. This led to the erroneous idea that traffic pollution was no longer a worry, as smog was less common. Then along came concerns about 'global warming' or climate change. The concern was that we had raised atmospheric concentrations of carbon dioxide enough to cause atmospheric temperatures to rise via the 'greenhouse effect', resulting in a catastrophic rise in global temperatures, the melting of the ice caps, and altered climate and weather patterns, resulting in global Armageddon. Thus in the late 1990s reducing atmospheric CO_2 levels and repairing the ozone became priorities.

Until recently most of the carbon dioxide in the air (concentration; 0.04 per cent) arose from geological weathering and respiration. Animal respiration contributed over many billions of years. Atmospheric carbon is in turn fixed by plants and sequestered by bodies of water and deposited into rocks as carbonates. This carbonate is locked away and buried below the earth's surface. The natural gas, coal and oil we burn to generate electricity, heat our homes and power our transport is all derived from the decomposed organic material: that is, dead animals, plants and microorganisms that were not recycled but buried beneath the surface. Global industrialization has led to the release of ever greater amounts of carbon dioxide into the atmosphere through burning these so-called fossil fuels. This industrial release is greater than the earth's natural ability to sequester the natural carbon dioxide being produced by today's geological weathering and life.

Thus, to reduce carbon dioxide emissions, diesel was championed over petrol as the amount of carbon exhausted into the air by diesel engines is lower than petrol-powered engines. This initiated a great switch to diesel engines. Diesel fuel and vehicles attracted less tax, and diesel-powered cars became the most popular vehicles promoted by all the world's car manufacturers. Of course, the streets were already full of large diesel-powered vehicles, such as lorries and buses. By the early twenty-first century it looked as if the petrol engine would become extinct. Nobody foresaw, or at least it was overlooked, that diesel fumes would create more air pollution, as these engines emit extra pollution in the form of very small particles of carbon into the air.

Diesel cars and taxis are the greatest contributors to traffic air pollution, accounting for around 35 per cent of the worldwide total. Diesel fuel does not burn as efficiently as petrol, so carbon particulates are produced. This can sometimes be seen as the black smoke that is expelled by exhaust pipes. Modern diesel vehicles do have filters to remove the larger smoke particles, but some of the smaller ones escape into the air, where they remain suspended. Someone breathing this air will inhale these microscopic particles deep into their lungs. Unfortunately, the wet environment of the lungs ensures that the particles are deposited rather than exhaled. These particles are called PM10, coarse particles, 2.5 to 10 microns in size, and PM2.5, fine particles, less than 2.5 microns in size, where a micron is a thousandth of a millimetre. Really small particles are called 'ultra-fine' or nanoparticles (a nanometre is a thousandth of a micron). These nanoparticles can pass into the blood and be transported and deposited around the body. The longer the exposure, the more particles accumulate in the lungs and tissues. In those who smoke, carbon particles (tar) from tobacco smoke are mixed in as well.

Following the introduction of unleaded petrol, all new cars were fitted with catalytic converters, allowing us to breathe less smoky air. Catalytic converters sit between the engine and the exhaust pipe. Their role is to reduce the noxious air-polluting gases produced by the engine. The converter consists of a simple ceramic and metal matrix through which the engine exhaust gases pass before being expelled through the rear exhaust or tailpipe. The metals in this matrix are platinum or aluminium and act as catalysts in combining the unburnt hydrogen and carbon from the fuel with carbon monoxide and oxygen from the air to produce carbon dioxide and water. The converters also reduce the nitrogen oxides (NOx) to nitrogen and carbon monoxide. They are not 100 per cent efficient, so some unconverted exhaust is expelled into the air. Without catalytic converters urban air would be noticeably unpleasant to breathe. Today, despite these converters, the increase in vehicle numbers has made NOx levels higher and more troublesome. They are now influencing people's health, particularly children, who are more vulnerable, and are thought to exacerbate respiratory disorders such as asthma. In sunny cloud-free weather the extra solar radiation creates ozone from this NOx, the ozone damaging the lungs further. For many urban-dwellers, breathing this air is unavoidable; it is tasteless, silent and invisible.

The recent Covid-19 pandemic has shown what happens when we remove traffic from the roads. Across the world air pollution levels have dropped drastically wherever there was a prolonged period of government-enforced home isolation.

Asthma and COPD are the main respiratory diseases affected by inhalation of vapours, gas, dust and fumes (known as VGDF). In the workplace there are many other respiratory diseases that result from VGDF exposure.[35] These include a wide range of less familiar respiratory diseases such as idiopathic pulmonary fibrosis (IPF), pulmonary alveolar proteinosis (PAP), hypersensitivity pneumonitis (HP), sarcoidosis and tuberculosis (TB). Breathing in flour dust at a bakery, or hay dust on a farm, leads to 'baker's lung' or 'baker's asthma', or 'farmer's lung'. Exposure to bird droppings and so on causes 'bird-fancier's lung' (psittacosis) and a variety of occupations such as paint spraying and metal welding can lead to lung disease and breathlessness. Some have only recently been described, such as berylliosis, caused by breathing in the metallic dust of elemental beryllium (Be). Its poisonous effects were not described until the 1940s, with one of the first victims being the American nuclear physicist Herbert L. Anderson, who was exposed to beryllium while working on the Manhattan Project.

While these particulates do not alter the way the majority of us breathe, chronic exposure can damage the deep recesses of the lung, especially the delicate, thin membranes where oxygen and carbon dioxide are exchanged between the air and blood. Today many people living near to roads and major transport arteries may in the future suffer respiratory illness as these particles slowly accumulate in their lungs. Breathing disorders are becoming more common in those living near traffic, especially children. It is has been proposed that schools near main roads should be closed or surrounded by trees, or the roads rerouted. With electric cars on the horizon, this problem will fade, but like all particulate matter, once these particles are breathed into the lungs and tissues, they remain there for life.

THE IDEAS OF miasma and the Victorian notion of hygienic ventilation no longer apply. We live in a world where draughts are excluded with double- or triple-glazed windows, close-fitting doors, and no open chimneys. Instead we breathe air that is 'conditioned', filtered and temperature-controlled. When we travel around our cities, we breathe NOx, ozone and particulates. Our burden of particulates and breathing 'bad air' has been reduced in some cases and increased in others. Tobacco smoking in public places has been banned in some countries, reducing our particulate loads. Naturally, our inhaled air is full of natural particles such as pollen, fungal spores, skin cells and dust, all of which we have lived with throughout time. While atmospheric carbon dioxide levels are too dilute to alter our breathing, it is its other chemical properties in trapping heat that are most lethal to humans. We are on a journey to reduce carbon pollution in the form of the two carbon gases carbon monoxide and carbon dioxide and now as carbonaceous particulate matter in the air from vehicle exhausts. Air pollution has become the greatest threat to the health of future generations.

After the Victorian era, breathing fresh air could no longer be taken for granted as society progressed from an agricultural to an industrial base. As urban populations exploded, clean air, once taken for granted, was now at a premium in big cities. The only places where fresh air can be found in plentiful supply are high in the atmosphere, the polar regions, the open sea and empty deserts. Living at high altitude presents many problems but humankind has slowly overcome these, and now millions of people live at higher elevations.

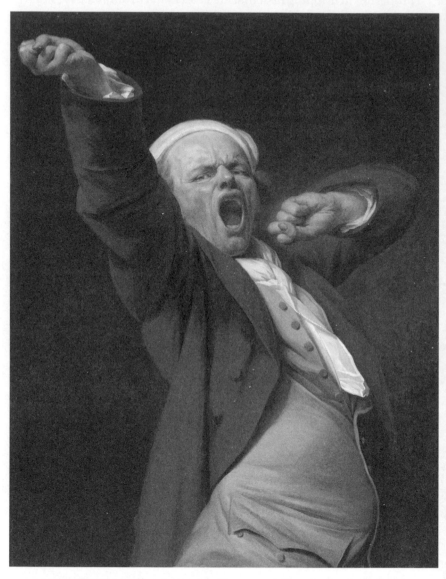

Joseph Ducreux, *Self-portrait*, 1783, oil on canvas. Yawning involves a large, slow inspiration with the mouth wide open and is often accompanied by stretching of the arms. It can also be contagious when observed.

FIVE

LABOURED BREATHING

B reathing is something we take for granted. We always feel at our best when we are breathing at a natural rhythm. There are, however, many occasions when this rhythm is disturbed. One such occasion is when we exert ourselves. We may huff and puff a little after climbing a flight of stairs, or pant heavily after running a short distance, but this sensation of being out of breath soon passes and usually within a minute or so our breathing returns to its normal slow rhythm. We subconsciously and quietly forget that it was ever an issue. At other times there is the embarrassing unguarded yawn at work or early in the morning queue at the coffee shop; again, this is a brief change in breathing, but nothing to worry about. However, there are many occasions when breathing becomes difficult and even life-threatening, in conditions such as polio, or disabling, in conditions such as COPD and obstructive sleep apnoea. Through the ingenuity of inventors and scientists, we have developed ways to aid and support our breathing, whether we are awake, asleep or unconscious. This is in sharp contrast to others who developed ways to hamper breathing, as in the use of gas weapons during the First World War.

Altered Breathing

One of the more distressing forms of arrhythmic breathing we all experience are hiccups. Brief episodes lasting a few minutes can be a little inconvenient, but longer bouts are another story and can affect personal well-being and even lead to social isolation. Loud hiccups can soon annoy a room full of people, be they colleagues, friends or family. Hiccupping can be very distracting and it is difficult to think of little else while experiencing them, so think how debilitating they must have been for Charles Osborne of Iowa, USA, who according to *Guinness World Records* hiccupped continuously for 68 years, starting in 1922 at the age of 28, when he suffered minor brain damage. He mysteriously stopped a year before his death in 1991.

In health, being breathless for a few minutes has little if any impact on your life, but in ill-health this is often not the case. You can become breathless even when motionless or after walking just a few yards. Unfortunately, breathlessness is a symptom of many medical conditions. In these conditions breathlessness or dyspnoea (its medical term from the Greek, meaning 'difficult breathing') is disabling and described by sufferers as air hunger, almost as if there is not enough air in the room anymore. It feels akin to suffocation – a severely unpleasant sensation unlike being out of breath due to simple exertion. Those who have experienced the sensation describe it differently: some complain of having to breathe too much, of not being able to breathe enough, of needing to take deep breaths, of gasping, suffocation or tightness in the chest or throat.[1]

Long-term or chronic breathlessness can be associated with lung disease and heart disease, so distinguishing the cause is not always straightforward. The most common lung condition where people report being breathless is COPD, which is a mixture of conditions, with the symptoms varying with severity. It is associated with smoking, and a debilitating breathlessness that becomes disabling in the severest cases, usually after many years of smoking. Smoking damages the structure of the lungs on a large scale, causing emphysema, where the lungs develop large pockets of empty space, which impedes oxygen transfer across the lungs into the blood. Often when the illness is severe, the COPD patient requires supplementary oxygen to breathe, even at rest. This can

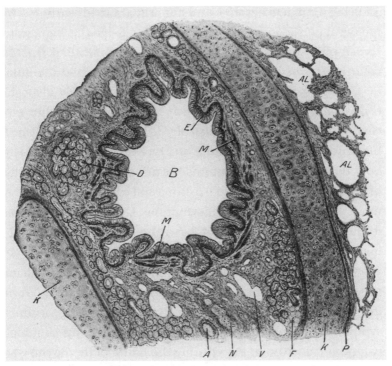

Cross-section through a small bronchus of a man (× 30), showing its semi-flexible shape. B, Bronchus, or airway, AL, alveoli, K, cartlidge, M, circular muscle, E, ciliated epithelium. Plate from the *Textbook of Histology* (1943).

be administered via a nasal mask or through two small prongs placed in the nose.

Asthma is another common respiratory disease in which the sufferers experience breathlessness. Today asthma can be self-managed by avoidance of triggers and taking inhaled medication. Asthma deaths in Europe have reduced markedly in the last thirty years, owing to better management of the disease. We now have a greater understanding of how to pharmacologically control the symptoms in the short and long term.[2] When asthma occurs in the young it is typically less deadly than asthma that appears in later life, when it is often associated with other complications such as COPD and heart disease.[3]

Asthma was known as far back as the second century BC, with the Greek physician Aretacus of Cappadocia from the first century

AD being the first to describe an asthma attack in his writings.[4] In medieval times Moses Maimonides (AD 1136–1204), a Sephardic Jewish philosopher, wrote a treatise on asthma called *Tractus contra passionem asthmatis*, in which he described the links between climate, diet and asthma. He was also an early advocate of clean air. Asthma was not seriously studied until the eighteenth century, when in 1769 the English physician John Millar published his *Observations on the Asthma and on the Hooping Cough*. His book defined the main symptoms, the principal being a 'difficulty of breathing'; he assumed that asthma and whooping cough (the modern name) shared similar symptoms. He dedicated his book to Queen Charlotte and stated that asthma was more of a childhood disease.

Another monarch mentioned in Millar's book is King William III (1650–1702), William of Orange, who suffered badly from asthma throughout his life. Millar stated that the king's asthma symptoms disappeared when a perpetually ulcerous shoulder wound he received in 1690 during the Battle of the Boyne was drained. At this time bloodletting was used as a cure for all ills, because bleeding was thought to restore the balance of the four humours. The wisdom at the time assigned asthma attacks to an imbalance in these humours.

As he aged, William sought to improve his asthma, so he and Queen Mary moved out of their swampy Westminster residence in London to Hampton Court Palace. In February 1702, while out riding his horse, he was violently thrown to the ground. The horse had stumbled on a fresh molehill, and on landing William broke his collarbone and was taken immediately to nearby Kensington Palace. Here he rested but unfortunately caught a chill, which slowly developed into pneumonia. He died aged 51 a few weeks later, on 8 March, his last recognizable words being 'I draw towards my end.' During his postmortem, his left lung was found to be full of a 'purulent frothy serum.'

Many neurological conditions alter breathing and are often accompanied by a sensation of breathlessness. In the lungs, when the nerves controlling the respiratory muscles are compromised, breathing is altered. This happens in the muscle-wasting disease muscular dystrophy. When the respiratory muscles degenerate and weaken, breathing becomes laboured. Death occurs through respiratory failure, when breathing is inadequate to maintain oxygenation, and ultimately the respiratory muscles fail and breathing stops. Another distressing condition is an acute neurological disorder known as Guillain-Barré syndrome (GBS), named after the French neurologists Georges Guillain, Jean-Alexandre Barré and André Strohl, who together first described the syndrome in two soldiers in 1916 while serving in the French Sixth Army during the First World War. The condition was diagnosed using cerebrospinal fluid sampled by lumbar puncture, the three doctors being early pioneers of this technique. The name of Strohl in time disappeared from the eponym.[5] The syndrome remained relatively obscure until the Second World War, when in the USA around fifty pathological specimens from fatal cases of GBS were brought together at the Armed Forces Institute of Pathology in Washington, DC. The specimens were collected from the many military hospitals scattered across the USA.

GBS is a rare autoimmune disorder in which the body attacks its own healthy nerves. It manifests quickly as a weakening of the muscles, beginning in the limbs with numbness and tingling, eventually leading to paralysis. In 25 per cent of cases the cranial nerve is affected, so that the patient requires ventilatory support to maintain their breathing. Often patients make a full recovery, but for around 10 per cent of sufferers it is fatal, with death resulting from respiratory complications.[6]

In some cases, the influenza virus has been suspected to be the cause of GBS. It was during the 1976–7 flu season that there was a huge spike in GBS numbers: around 1,100 cases were reported in the USA alone. At the beginning of 1976, a 'swine flu' was expected to arrive later in the year, so during the latter months, 45 million doses of influenza vaccine were administered to the public. With the sudden appearance of the 1,100 cases of GBS, a link with the vaccine was identified, so it was quickly withdrawn and no more GBS cases appeared. Despite this rapid response, there was a great public outcry once it was known that the vaccine could potentially have been a fatal cause of GBS. This led to 4,000 legal actions being filed against the U.S. federal government demanding a total of $3 billion in damages. The Department of Justice defended the legal action, and, in the end, claimants were compensated for the cost of the illness only. This reduced the government's compensation costs to the tens of millions of dollars. No one doubts that there was a spike in cases of GBS during this period, but it remains unclear as to whether this was caused by the vaccine or was pure coincidence. Even today, despite the evidence that vaccination is safe and provides complete protection from numerous diseases, a small number of the public remain sceptical, thus ensuring that the infection rates remain high enough to perpetuate the spread of viruses; this has prevented the elimination of the common measles or polio viruses, for example.

The British Labour party politician Anthony Neil Wedgwood Benn (1925–2014), better known as Tony Benn, suffered and survived GBS while in his fifties, during a particularly politically turbulent time within the Labour Party. His subsequent hospitalization was sudden, and some believed he had been poisoned. He had to suspend his political career for three months. This single bout of GBS left him slightly deaf for the rest of his life and sometimes affected his balance, which made him stagger. To the casual observer, this could be mistaken for drunkenness (although he was a teetotaller). Despite this, his career continued and he died aged 88.

People who suffer injuries or trauma to their brainstems can often need artificial ventilation to breathe because their respiratory muscles are paralysed. In some cases, after a few days or weeks, as the person slowly regains consciousness, they are still quadriplegic and lack the ability to consciously control their breathing but still retain the ability to breathe spontaneously without a ventilator. This is because they still have automatic control (central) but not voluntary control (peripheral) of their breathing; they are voiceless, as this requires voluntary control.

Often the only way to communicate is by eye movements (up or down) or eyelid blinks (for example, with one blink for yes and two for no). This condition was given a name in 1966 by Fred Plum and Jerome B. Posner, who called it 'locked-in syndrome' (LIS), or pseudocoma.[7] The condition was known before this and the first medical paper describing LIS was published in 1875 by the French physician M. Darolles, although its description had appeared in the well-known novel *The Count of Monte Cristo* by Alexandre Dumas (1844–5). In this novel the character Monsieur Noirtier de Villefort is depicted as 'a corpse with living eyes', and communicates by blinking.[8]

People with LIS have used this form of optical communication to write entire books, the most famous, perhaps, being *The Diving-bell and the Butterfly* (1997), by French journalist Jean-Dominique Bauby. The loss of the ability to consciously control breathing is apparent in other neural conditions, such as the slowly progressing amyotrophic lateral sclerosis (ALS) suffered by the famous English physicist Stephen Hawking (1942–2018), who communicated using a now iconic computerized voice.

Disordered Sleep

A good night's sleep is important, for without it our physical and mental health deteriorate. We cannot do without sleep, as it fulfils many functions, both physiological and psychological. While we sleep our conscious minds become detached and we enter a semi-comatose state where we seem to be unaware of our surroundings while retaining the subconscious ability to notice changes in our environment. We have all experienced waking suddenly from sleep, sometimes with a start, even though the room is dark and quiet, and for no apparent reason, while at other times you might wake to the telephone ringing or a clap of thunder. In either case, you gasp as you awaken and take a few rapid breaths. The brain remains active during sleep, supporting our vital functions, such as maintaining blood pressure and breathing. Throughout the night our sleep passes through several stages, each of a different depth and duration. When in deep sleep, breathing is slow, shallow and regular, and occurs quietly through the nose (the mouth being shut). While asleep, the breathing cycle differs to the cycle seen while awake. The sleeper's breath begins with a short sharp inspiration (as the diaphragm contracts) and a short sharp expiration (as the diaphragm relaxes), followed by a short, relaxed pause when nothing happens before the next breath begins. When awake, the expiratory pause is usually missing.

When breathing is disrupted, either by the airways becoming narrowed or by periods of no breathing (called apnoea), the amount of oxygen in the blood drops quickly while the amount of CO_2 rises, which causes further disturbances in breathing. Sleep-disordered breathing is quite common in elderly people. Obstructive sleep apnoea (OSA) is the most common presentation of this disorder and is most frequently found in men who are overweight. Men often deposit extra weight around their necks, a form of weight gain that is less common in women. In OSA, when sleeping lying down, the upper pharynx, the throat, collapses, and the tongue falls backwards; this narrows the upper airway (throat), and the person then switches from nose breathing to mouth breathing, which can be noisy and can generate snoring. Under mild conditions this snoring is undetected and does not have serious outcomes. As the obstruction gets worse the snoring gets worse and periods of apnoea develop. The sleeper may not realize that their breathing is so irregular and awake feeling tired, often falling asleep again during quiet moments. For those whose employment involves driving, this can be very dangerous. Many OSA sufferers seek medical advice only after waking suddenly from 'microsleeps' while driving. Many fatal crashes result from unrecognized OSA. The long-term solution is to change lifestyle, be active, eat sensibly and lose weight. Weight loss, particularly around the neck, restores normal pharyngeal airflow and the snoring stops. In the short-term, mechanical ventilation while asleep can be used, known as non-invasive ventilation. The person with OSA wears a tight-fitting mask over their nose and mouth while they sleep. The ventilator detects each expiration and maintains a slight positive pressure in the throat until inspiration begins, when the ventilator provides air. This positive pressure helps to hold or splint the airways open.

Some people with OSA, around 10–20 per cent, suffer from another condition that alters daytime breathing, called obesity hypoventilation syndrome (OHS). In OHS any excess upper body weight makes breathing more difficult. Thus someone with OHS experiences not only sleep-disordered breathing, such as OSA, but chronic daytime hypoventilation, which leads to sleepiness, snoring and excess salivation. The sleepiness is associated with high carbon dioxide levels in the blood.[9] Constantly falling asleep during the day leads to a poor quality of life. One OHS patient was observed falling asleep while standing on a doorstep just waiting for a door to be answered.[10] This condition is well known today, but its vague symptoms were not recognized as a medical condition fully until 1969. The first published report of someone with obesity and hypersomnolence (sleepiness) was in 1889, reported by a Dr R. Canton as a 'Case of narcolepsy'; the patient in question was a poulter from Liverpool who often fell asleep while serving customers at the counter, only to wake fifteen minutes later still holding the duck or chicken. He could not sit down without falling asleep, even when he went to the theatre, a favourite pastime. He even fell asleep while carving a joint at the table. His condition improved greatly after he lost weight.

The excessive daytime sleepiness is not due to tiredness but to inadequate breathing. With OHS the amount of carbon dioxide in the blood builds while the amount of oxygen falls.[11] Thus the person moves more towards coma than sleep, with loud snoring and nocturnal choking.

The syndrome was finally recognized by the American physician Charles Sidney Burwell and his Harvard colleagues in 1956, who named the condition 'Pickwickian syndrome' after a character in Charles Dickens's first novel, *The Posthumous Papers of the Pickwick Club* (1836). The character in question is Mr Wardle's servant Joe, an obese young man who throughout the book is always falling asleep and must be woken up. Joe appears several times in the story and serves to provide a vivid description of this condition, pre-dating the clinical case study of 1889.

> Mr Wardle unconsciously changed the subject, by calling emphatically for Joe.
> 'Damn that boy,' said the old gentleman, 'he's gone to sleep again.'
> 'Very extraordinary boy that,' said Mr Pickwick; 'does he always sleep in this way?'
> 'Sleep!' said the old gentleman, 'He's always asleep. Goes on errands fast asleep, and snores as he waits at table.'
> 'How very odd!' said Mr Pickwick.
> 'Ah! odd indeed,' returned the old gentleman; 'I'm proud of that boy – wouldn't part with him on any account – he's a natural curiosity!'

Before being ascribed to breathing, obesity and somnolence, a condition best described by pulmonary medicine, Joe's condition was considered to be endocrine in origin, perhaps due to hypothyroidism, hypopituitarism (Froehlich's syndrome) or even dystrophia adiposogenitalis, a growth deficiency disorder.

One condition that is exceedingly rare, but more deadly than OHS, is central hypoventilation syndrome (CHS), which alters breathing when sleeping and can occur in neonates and adults. When it is present in the newborn it is called primary CHS. In both cases the child or adult is unable to match their breathing rate or ventilation with their blood oxygen and carbon dioxide levels, as the sensing mechanism is abnormal or damaged. In the congenital primary CHS form it is thought to be due to an altered gene called PHOX-2B. In adults CHS manifests through damage to the sensing mechanisms via disease such as poliomyelitis or trauma. People with CHS often need to use a mechanical ventilator while they sleep, as they cannot support their breathing unconsciously, running the risk of stopping breathing altogether while asleep and dying from asphyxiation. In the daytime their breathing can be supported by a 'breathing pacemaker', similar to a cardiac pacemaker, but instead of stimulating the cardiac muscle, it stimulates the diaphragm, the main breathing muscle.

Although deaths from this condition have occurred since ancient times, they went unnoticed until the first medical reports appeared in 1955. Its cause was not determined until 1962, when two Americans, the anaesthetist John Severinghaus and the physician Robert A. Mitchell, described three patients who had difficulty breathing even while awake. They coined the name 'Ondine's curse' for the disorder (although calling it a curse might be considered a bit too dramatic). Severinghaus had recently seen the play *Ondine*. The plot originated from an old folk tale of a water nymph known as Undine, which has been told in many forms as a popular story. In the original myth Ondine meets and falls in love with a mortal, Hans, a knight errant whom she marries against the advice of her fellow nymphs. Ondine discovers that her husband prefers his original love, a mortal woman, Bertha. Ondine curses Hans so that he cannot rest, telling him that if he forgets her, he will die. So, the idea is that a person who has Ondine's curse will similarly die if they forget to breathe.

In young babies the inability to match breathing with blood oxygen and carbon dioxide levels during sleep can also lead to sudden infant death syndrome (SIDS) and sudden unexplained death in epileptics.[12]

As adults, we breathe freely and easily because our thorax is free to expand rhythmically with each breath. We consciously avoid wearing tight clothing that restricts the chest as it makes breathing more difficult. The effect on breathing of tight clothing can be seen in the corset. Originally called a 'quilted waistcoat', the corset became popular for both men and women in the early nineteenth century. In women the corset was used to give the wearer an hourglass figure and extended from under the breasts to the waist. The whalebone stays, when laced tight, could not be over-tightened and hamper breathing. Later the whalebone was replaced with steel stays and the invention of iron-eyelets allowed the lacing to be pulled tighter and tighter. Many a fashionable

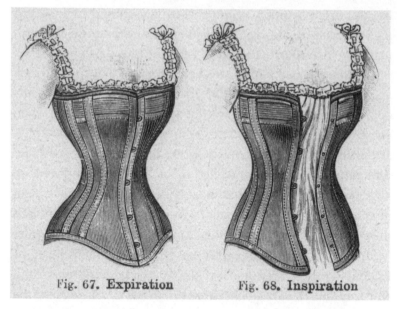

Fig. 67. Expiration   Fig. 68. Inspiration

While the corset provided a slim waist, it also impeded breathing by
compressing the abdomen. Illustration from Anna Fischer, *La femme,
medecin du foyer*, c. 1900.

young lady would faint owing to an inability to breathe sufficiently,
as the overtight corset restricted movement of the chest and
abdomen. Many large houses of the time contained 'fainting
rooms', private rooms to which corseted women could retire if
they were overcome by faintness. Sometimes, if worn from an
early age, the corset could restrict growth and even lead to
reduced fertility. While today most people would consider this
degree of compression unhealthy, at that time the view was split:
some medical professionals thought it healthy and others did
not. The medical journal *The Lancet*, which published case studies such as 'Death from Tight Lacing' in 1890, reports the death
of a Berlin theatre actress thought to be due to an overtight corset,
and warns of 'these foolish persons whose false taste and vanity
have made them suffering devotees of a custom so injurious'.

Two years later, *The Lancet* report 'Effects of Tight-lacing'
described the distorted thorax and abdomen of a fifty-year-old
woman, who was believed to have died from wearing her corset
too tight. Eventually the tight-laced corset became unpopular.

Wearing one was not only seen as unhealthy but as a sign of moral indecency. In the Edwardian era the corset became softer and eventually evolved into the girdle, which did not restrict breathing in any serious way.

Heavy Breathing and Asphyxia

While a tight corset may restrict breathing, if the chest is restricted for a prolonged period then death ensues. Unfortunately, history is littered with many tragic occasions where multiple deaths from compression asphyxia occurred. One of the most notorious cases of mass compression asphyxia occurred on 20 June 1756 in Calcutta (now Kolkata), India, when 146 British soldiers and their wives were captured and held captive in a small guardroom overnight. The unfortunate event became known as the Black Hole of Calcutta and resulted in 123 people dying of asphyxiation. The room was 6.7 metres by 4.6 metres (22 by 15 ft), unlit and poorly ventilated by two small windows. The ambient temperature was hot (34°C, or 93°F) and the captives soon started to complain of dehydration. As the night wore on, some of the captives lost consciousness and fell to the floor, where they were stepped upon by their still-standing fellow captives. As more people fainted, those already lying on the floor were crushed further. By the morning only those close to the open windows had survived. The senior officer John Zephaniah Holwell, who was near a window and survived the ordeal, later wrote a detailed account of the night. He managed to remain hydrated by drinking the moisture and sweat captured in his shirt sleeves. Unfortunately, this did not work for the other captives as they removed their shirts because of the heat.[13]

A less well-known but equally horrifying case of mass compression asphyxia is the Victoria Hall disaster that occurred on Saturday, 16 June 1883, in Sunderland, Tyne and Wear, in which 183 young children died. On the day around 1,100 children were crammed into the hall to watch a free magic and puppet show. The event was made all the more popular, for each child was promised a gift upon leaving the event. The organizers decided to distribute the gifts outside the hall and when the show ended directed the children up some stairs to a back corridor, which ended in stairs down to a backdoor exit. The children had to queue down a stairway before leaving through a large inward-opening door. When the show ended, the unsupervised children, excited from the show and keen to collect their gifts, rushed up the stairs. When the first children reached the exit door, it was jammed only partially open. As the excited children surged down the stairs, a child got stuck in the partially opened door, and became tangled with the other children trying to push through. The doorway quickly became impassable and those behind the door had nowhere to go and soon became trapped. Unaware of this, the children in the upper corridor continued surging forwards, pushing those at the top of the stairs, who fell onto those at the bottom. The pile of fallen children quickly increased and those at the bottom of the pile were crushed and unable to breathe. Eventually the adults in the hall realized what was happening and prevented further deaths by turning the five hundred or so children in the upstairs corridor back to the hall. At the back door the adults furiously pulled those trapped out through the partially open door. The tragedy was a national disaster and reported nationwide with great abhorrence. The event was followed by two public enquiries and no one was found to be responsible for the disaster. However, Parliament did enact new laws requiring that all places of public entertainment should have numerous exit doors that open outwards. The hall was eventually destroyed in April 1941 by a German air raid and never rebuilt.

Cases of mass compression asphyxiation still occur. In April 1999, overcrowding at a Nottingham Forest versus Liverpool football match at Hillsborough Stadium in Sheffield led to 96 deaths. Too many people had been let into the stadium and a crush started from the entering fans filling the stands from the rear. On one stand where the Liverpool supporters gathered to watch the game, the pressure became too much, and the crowd collapsed forwards. The pitch side was fenced off, so those at the bottom of the stands had nowhere to escape to. The tragedy unfolded as the emergency services struggled to reach the crushed spectators, which included adults and children.

Today, panic engendered by fire or fire alarms continues to lead to death from compression asphyxia, especially in over-crowded nightclubs and discos, where personal closeness is part of the experience. When deaths occur, it is usually due to the fire doors being blocked intentionally in order to prevent people from getting in without paying or queuing at the front.

When breathing has been prevented or stopped for a few minutes, it can sometimes be restored by mouth-to-mouth resuscitation or expired air ventilation (EAV). Mouth-to-mouth describes the manoeuvre in which the lungs of an unconscious person are forcefully inflated by a bystander (such as a rescuer or paramedic) exhaling into their mouth by pressing their mouth against the mouth of the unconscious victim. This manoeuvre is used to force the victim to breathe. This works especially well if they have been recovered from the water after submersion and their lungs are waterlogged. EAV can also be combined with cardiac compressions, an emergency technique known as CPR (cardiopulmonary resuscitation). CPR involves rhythmically pressing down on the breastbone (sternum), while intermittently inflating the lungs using EAV. This will in many cases restart the heart if the victim has fainted owing to the heart stopping. This is not to be confused with cardioversion, a technique which uses a defibrillator, a device which stops the irregularly beating heart altogether via an electrical jolt applied to the chest. This allows the heart to spontaneously restart again, generally with a regular rhythm. The purpose of all of these manoeuvres is to ensure that the brain and heart remain adequately supplied with oxygen. Once breathing and the blood are moving again, recovery begins and the person usually regains consciousness.

The ability to stimulate breathing by expelling air into someone's lungs was first reported therapeutically in 1732 in Alloa, Scotland, by the local surgeon William Tossach, who revived a miner, James Blair, who had been brought up lifeless from the pit.[14] Tossach describes how he 'blowed my breath as strong as I could'.

James soon began breathing again and his pulse could shortly be felt at his wrist. He recovered fully.

The history of mouth-to-mouth resuscitation is thought by many to begin with a description in the Old Testament in 2 Kings 4:32–5, where the prophet Elisha revives an unconscious Shunammite child by inflating their lungs.[15] The text is vague about how this was achieved and does not specify that mouth-to-mouth resuscitation was used. Therefore it does not fit our modern view of EAV. At the time it was seen more as a miracle, a transfer of the life force, pneuma, found in the breath.

On many occasions members of the public have revived unconscious people by using EAV. From medieval times EAV was used by midwives to resuscitate newborn babies. By far the commonest use was to resuscitate someone after drowning. EAV was

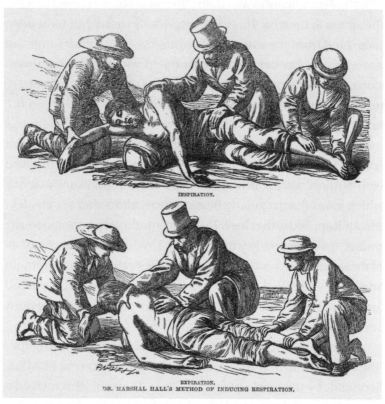

INSPIRATION.

EXPIRATION.
DR. MARSHAL HALL'S METHOD OF INDUCING RESPIRATION.

Dr Marshall Hall's method for resuscitating a drowned person, 1864. Here the person is rotated, the movement stimulating respiration using gravity.

frowned upon, however, as it was considered degrading to touch those who had died an 'unnatural death'.[16] This view was changed by the creation of humane societies set up by wealthy philanthropists across Europe and the USA. The first such society was the Society for the Recovery of Drowned Persons, established in 1767 in Amsterdam. It was founded to inform the public about using mouth-to-mouth resuscitation to revive the many people who fell in the city's canals. The society, and the implementation of mouth-to-mouth resuscitation, was successful in saving 150 lives in its first four years. By the eighteenth century the commonest form of accidental death in the UK was from drowning.[17] In 1774 London followed Amsterdam with its own institute named 'An Institution for affording Immediate Relief to Persons Apparently Dead from Drowning', later to become the Humane Society.

While mouth-to-mouth was considered suitable for the layperson to resuscitate the drowning, the medical profession had to deal with various causes of asphyxia, or, as it was termed then, 'suspended animation', which included 'drowning, hanging, noxious vapours, syncope or lightning strikes and unborn children surviving the death of their mothers'. For these cases it was recommended to use tubes and bellows, as mouth-to-mouth was considered too 'vulgar'. For this reason, it lost its popularity among the medical profession and by the 1840s the Humane Society dismissed artificial ventilation as of secondary importance.[18] Thus during the nineteenth century mouth-to-mouth was almost forgotten. The Royal Humane Society advocated a technique where the unconscious person was revived by alternatively turning them onto their left and right sides while returning them to their back in between, the so-called ready method.

President Abraham Lincoln was a recipient of mouth-to-mouth resuscitation. On Good Friday 1865, 14 April, Lincoln was assassinated by being shot in the head. The young doctor Charles Leale is said to have applied mouth-to-mouth breathing, restoring Lincoln's breathing for long enough for him to be moved to a hotel, where he died the next morning at 7.20 a.m. There is some doubt this ever happened as Leale did not report his experience until 44 years later in 1909, at an event celebrating the centenary of Lincoln's birth.

Mouth-to-mouth resuscitation was advocated in the 1940s by the u.s. Coast Guard Service and the Chicago, Detroit and Los Angeles fire departments, who would provide mouth-to-mouth resuscitation until medical help arrived. It was not until the 1950s that mouth-to-mouth resuscitation was combined with CPR, when it became acceptable again. By the 1960s it formed part of the recommendations for basic life support using A-B-C (Airways, Breathing and Circulation).

Mechanical Breathing

During the period when mouth-to-mouth resuscitation was unpopular, many ingenious physicians, engineers and inventors came up with a variety of solutions to revive the unconscious person. While some developed alternative manoeuvres, others developed bellows and tubes. These contraptions were designed to ventilate or support the person for only short periods of time, as natural breathing was expected to return within 15–30 minutes at the most. Any longer than this and mechanical ventilation would permanently damage the lungs, as often too much pressure was used to inflate them. This left room for more inventive physicians such as John Dalziel, of Drumlanrig, Scotland, who in 1832 published his essay 'On Sleep and an Apparatus for Promoting Artificial Ventilation' describing his invention of the first tank respirator.[19] As the name suggests, the patient to be ventilated is placed in an airtight box while the air pressure in the box is cycled from atmospheric pressure to sub-atmospheric pressure, causing the lungs to inflate and deflate. Thus the breathing rate and depth could be controlled by bellows and valves. While this worked, it was impractical in allowing access to and was claustrophobic for the patient. In later versions the patient's head was covered in a tight elastic cap with the face left uncovered.

In 1880 the Austrian physician, Dr Ignez von Hauke (1832–1885) at Crown Prince Joseph's Children's Hospital in Vienna prolonged a girl's life for three months by giving her respiratory support for 2–3 hours per day using his tank respirator or *pneumatische Apparate*.[20] Hauke went on to develop another device to assist breathing, which he called the *pneumatischer Panzer* or pneumatic tank, from the French word *pancier*, a breastplate. This class of device became known as a cuirass, a word that dates back to the fifteenth century and also refers to the breastplate, a piece of armour covering the chest. Hauke's device is like a miniature tank that just encompasses the thorax, and makes patient look as if they are wearing a giant tortoise shell on their front. A cuirass works by cycling negative pressure around the chest, allowing atmospheric air to inflate the lungs and actively supporting inhalation. Exhalation is passive and brought about by releasing the negative pressure and restoring the cuirass pressure back to atmospheric pressure, which allows the lungs to deflate.

Over the nineteenth century various improvements were made to both tank and cuirass devices, with great inventors such as Alexander Graham Bell contributing to the technology. By 1908, Peter Lord of Worcester, Massachusetts, had patented a whole respirator room with two large pistons in the ceiling creating the required pressure changes. The whole contrivance was too expensive and never got built.

The technology continued advancing slowly as a specialist area of intensive care and supporting a small number of patients. For drowning victims, the technology developed in parallel in France. Alfred Woillez built the first workable lung fabricated from iron instead of wood, which he named the Spirophore, in 1876. He proposed that these iron box ventilators should be placed along the River Seine, so that they would be immediately available to help people who had drowned.[21]

As the 1900s progressed, the demand for artificial respiratory support was to grow dramatically. Poliomyelitis, a highly contagious viral disease often caught in childhood, frequently led to paralysis and incapacitation. Paralysis of the limbs was common, but often it could result in the gradual paralysis of the respiratory muscles, eventually leading to death. Around the world

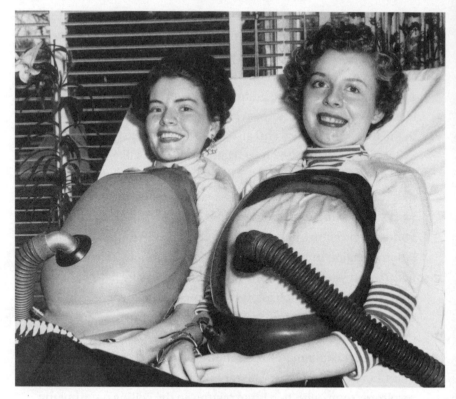

Two polio victims using cuirass ventilators in 1955. Negative pressure is generated inside the sealed ventilator shell, which allows the lungs to inflate (inspiration). This is followed by the application of a positive pressure, facilitating expiration.

hospitals could be overwhelmed by local epidemics. It was the tank respirator that came to the rescue. The first person to attempt to use the tank respirator to treat his patients was Dr W. Steuart of South Africa, in 1918, who during an epidemic designed his own version with an electric motor to drive the pressure pumps. Unfortunately, all of his patients died before he managed to build his first device. The important but subtle advance was that he had designed a negative pressure ventilator that could support respiration indefinitely, as the electric pumps took away the need for manual pumping.

The first successes came in 1928 when three members of Harvard Medical School published two papers describing a tank ventilator. These ventilators soon became known as the 'iron lung'. The authors were Philip Drinker, an engineer, Charles F. McKhann, a paediatrician, and Louis Agassiz Shaw, a physiologist. The tank, now a sheet metal cylinder, enclosed the patient, whose head and neck protruded through a sealed collar. The pressure inside the chamber was changed using commercial electric vacuum cleaner motors, in this case from the Electric Blower company in Boston.[22] These were the first commercially produced tank respirators. In 1930 Drinker brought his tank respirator to the UK, where it was then known in the medical profession as a mechanical respirator, but dubbed by *The Times* newspaper the 'iron lung', a term still familiar to many people today. Sir Robert Davis bought the ventilator with a view to manufacturing it in the UK. While the design was simplified, the original ventilator was lent to several hospitals, where it was used to save lives. The UK version of the Drinker respirometer was ready by 1934 and cost around £97 (approximately £5,000 today).[23]

In Australia, the limited number of Drinker respirators in use were saving lives. The respirators were imported from the USA and proved expensive and difficult to maintain. When the respirators broke, they had to be repaired in the factory back in the USA, so sending them back and forth was inconvenient. In 1937 there was a polio epidemic in Adelaide and too few ventilators to support the patients. This led to the South Australian Health Department asking the brother engineers Edward and Donald Both to design a cheap alternative. In the physics department at the University of Adelaide they built their Both respirators, in which the patient was placed in a sealed wooden cabinet or tank. Being wooden, this respirator was much cheaper, quicker to build and lighter to transport. Edward Both had already established the medical instrument company Both Equipment Ltd in order to sell other devices he had earlier designed and made, including an early ECG recorder. His devices were popular in Australia, but it was a limited market, so he decided to promote his instruments and organized a world business trip. While in the UK in 1938, Both and his wife heard a BBC radio appeal for a Drinker ventilator to save a boy with polio. Both instantly went to work. Some accounts say

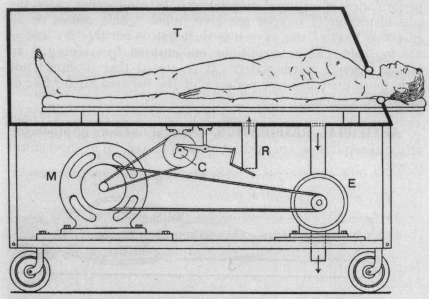

FIG. 79.—Drinker's artificial respiration apparatus.
T. = Airtight tank.   E = Exhaust fan.   M. = Motor.
R. = Release valve.   C. = Cam.

Drinker artificial respiration apparatus, or iron lung. The patient lies in a coffin-shaped box (T) with their heading protruding through a sealed collar. The air pressure inside the box is cycled between negative and atmosphric by the motor (M),thus supporting ventilation. Illustration from Bainbridge and Menzie's *Essentials of Physiology* (1936).

that he built a respirator right there in his rented flat, but it is more likely that he hired a workshop and built several. One of these was featured in a film on the subject created by the Nuffield Department of Anaesthetics at the University of Oxford, based at the Radcliffe Infirmary, the first academic anaesthetics department in the world. It had been founded by William Morris (ennobled as Viscount Nuffield in 1938), who was the owner of Morris Motors Limited, which produced many thousands of cars, such as the Morris Ten. Nuffield saw this film and was immediately impressed by the device, planning to build them at his Morris Motor works at Cowley, Oxford.

Lord Nuffield's involvement changed the field. In 1938 there were 32 Drinker respirators in the whole of the UK, but by March

1939 there were 669 Both respirators. This was a vast improvement but lower than the target of 5,000 that Nuffield had planned.

This rapid emergence of cheap respirators created some controversy and a correspondence grew in the medical press. Some of the medical profession were all for the technology but others were cautious. The target of 5,000 instruments was questioned, as it was pointed out that it was early days and little was known about the technology. They could soon become useless if modifications were needed, and if distributed widely to hospitals, the hospital staff would not know how to use them. In the end, five hundred more iron lungs were proposed instead.[24] Schemes to train staff and the setting up of specialist centres were proposed, but they did not help, as Lord Nuffield advocated mass production while the medical profession, particularly Sir Frederick Menzies and Sir Leonard Hill, rallied against him. It turns out that both were right. In 1939 a Dr H. N. Garrus wrote,

> We have two cockerels in the roost, Business acumen represented by Lord Nuffield and professional wisdom represented by Sir Frederick Menzies and his friends. Rather than goad them into fighting we should encourage them to get together for the good of all.[25]

The NHS soon adopted the notion of keeping costs down by bulk buying. By the beginning of the Second World War there were many thousands of iron lungs around the world.[26]

Supported breathing by the iron lung depended on negative pressure ventilation, which was opposite to positive pressure ventilation, as in mouth-to-mouth resuscitation or bellows-assisted breathing. The problem with positive pressure ventilation is that if it is applied too vigorously, it can overinflate the lungs and cause damage by too much pressure (causing barotrauma) or too large a volume (volutrauma), so it was only used for short periods.

The watershed moment for using positive pressure ventilation was sparked by a polio epidemic. The epidemic is thought to have originated in attendees of the World Polio Congress in

Copenhagen, Denmark, in 1951. The following summer, a polio epidemic appeared in Copenhagen, with around fifty polio patients being admitted to Blegdams Infectious Hospital. The mortality rate was around 87 per cent, and no one really knew why, although kidney failure was suspected as the cause of death. However, an anaesthetist, Bjorn Ibsen, thought it might be respiratory failure. Ibsen, at first unsupported by others in the field, proved his views by ventilating the patients with positive pressure ventilation and dramatically reduced the death rate to 40 per cent. The one big problem with this approach at the time was that the ventilators had to be manually operated and squeezed by hand. These consisted of a flexible reservoir and a one-way valve, so that when the reservoir bag was squeezed it emptied fresh air into a face mask, which, when placed firmly over the patient's mouth and nose, would force air into the lungs. When the reservoir bag was released the positive pressure in the lungs would allow the lungs to deflate naturally back to their resting volume. In the meantime, the deflated bag would refill with fresh air, ready to be

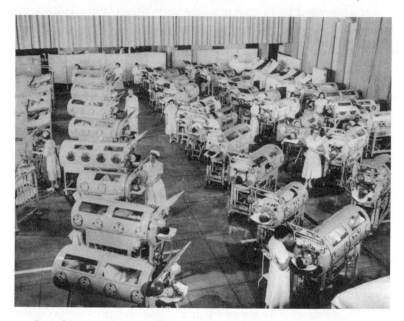

Over thirty iron-lung respirators were used at the Rancho Los Amigos Respirator Center in Hondo, California, to treat paralysed polio patients during the u.s. epidemic of 1952–3.

squeezed again for the next breath. Supporting breathing this way requires the operator to repeat this manoeuvre about 6–10 times a minute. Reservoir squeezing has to be done at just the right rate and volume so as not to cause barotrauma or volutrauma, and not too infrequently, as this would lead to the supply of oxygen being insufficient. Too quick, and gas exchange would become inefficient. Thus during the polio epidemic, to continuously ventilate all the patients, shifts of 'baggers' would be required, each person 'bagging' a patient for a few hours at a time. In the Blegdams Hospital the problem was not the bagging, but sheer numbers. At the peak of the epidemic they had seventy patients requiring ventilation. To meet this demand an army of medical students, 1,500 in all, was recruited, who between them supplied 165,000 hours of manual ventilation. At the time, the global impact of this exercise on the medical profession was immense. This event has been eclipsed recently by the work required to ventilate patients with Covid-19, where oxygen delivery by mask, respirator or ventilator was essential in treating the many thousands who globally succumbed to the infection.

Treating so many polio patients successfully showed that positive pressure ventilation could replace breathing in people requiring intensive care. Since then, the technology has come of age and the side-effects have slowly been overcome. Raised pressure alone is not a problem; after all, trumpet players generate high lung pressures while playing and suffer little lung damage. It is the way the breath is delivered in terms of pressure and volume that needs to be carefully controlled. The inspired breath must build slowly rather than all at once. When an unconscious person is ventilated in an intensive care unit (ICU) breathing occurs via a stiff plastic tube inserted into the trachea, which traverses the vocal cords.

Theses endotracheal tubes (ET tube) are necessary to ensure that the mechanical breath is passed only to the lungs and not down into the stomach, for instance. On the end of each ET tube is an inflatable cuff that, once inflated, blocks the space surrounding the tube and therefore seals the trachea, preventing

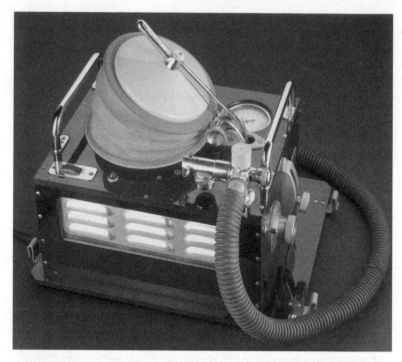

An early portable ventilator. Air or oxygen was delivered to the patient via a rubber concertina reservoir bag, which was regularly compressed by a small electric motor. The bedside ventilator initiated the development of the intensive care ward, as more and more sophisticated monitoring equipment was created from the 1950s onwards.

air leaking backwards from the lungs, especially when the lungs are fully inflated. To place the ET tube in the trachea, a procedure called intubation, is quite tricky. Intubation requires a special instrument called a laryngoscope to be inserted in the throat. This device has a long, slightly curved blade (those used for adult airways are about 15 cm (6 in.) long), which is blunt and has a small light embedded in the end. Once inserted into the throat, it allows the operator to flatten the tongue and raise the epiglottis, bringing into view the vocal cords and glottis and allowing the ET tube to be guided down the blade and pushed through the vocal cords into the trachea before the balloon is inflated. This is usually performed while the patient is anaesthetized but can also be performed in emergencies when the person is unconscious and not breathing properly.

Before its invention in the early 1940s by the New Zealand-born anaesthetist Sir Robert Reynolds Macintosh, the first professor of the Nuffield Department of Anaesthetics at the University of Oxford, laryngoscopes were not widely used. Intubation was only sometimes successful, as the anaesthetist had to blindly push the ET tube through the mouth or nose. Macintosh had commercial connections with the medical instrument industry, and the leading American anaesthetic equipment manufacturer Foregger promoted the device aggressively. Today the Macintosh laryngoscope is used worldwide.[27] The Foregger company, founded by Richard von Foregger, no longer exists as the company's influence waned in the late 1950s, principally because its founder refused to adopt newer innovations made by young up-and-coming anaesthetists, who in their frustration created rival companies, which ultimately became more successful. The company was dissolved in 1987.[28] Modern ventilators are much gentler on the lungs and can keep people ventilated for many years.

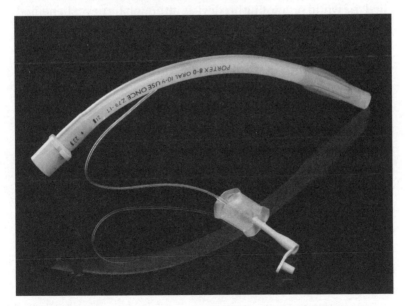

An endotracheal tube is inserted into the lung trachea usually via the mouth. After the tube has been inserted the cuff is inflated, which anchors the tube and provides an airtight seal. This allows the lungs to be inflated with positive pressure and ensures oxygen delivery. The top of the tube is connected to a ventilator.

The story of supported breathing does not end here. The ET tube was greatly improved by the British anaesthesiologist Archie Ian Jeremy Brain, who, working alone at home and at the Royal London Hospital in the 1980s, invented the first prototype laryngeal mask.[29] This is a shorter tube with a soft inflatable mask on the end which sits over the larynx. Once inflated, it seals the airway from the oesophagus, protecting the lungs and allowing easier mechanical breathing. Thus, unlike the ET tube, it does not need to be inserted into the trachea or windpipe. After trying it on himself, Brain next used it on a patient in 1981, doing so without any permission whatsoever. After further research, this time with ethical consent but still working alone, he developed improved versions, soon inserting the device in around 7,000 patients. In 1983 he finally attracted some funding and the mask became commercially available in 1989. After this its use rose meteorically, with over 100 million patients being intubated with the device worldwide by 1995. Brain's life changed dramatically, and he travelled the world promoting his device, although he never benefited greatly from his invention financially.

Many people with obstructive sleep apnoea will be familiar with another form of mechanical ventilation known as NIPPV, which supports a treatment known as CPAP or continuous positive airway pressure. CPAP is not delivered by an ET tube or laryngeal mask but by a tightly fitting mask nestled over the nose. More importantly, it is applied while the person is fully conscious, but is usually worn when the person sleeps. It supports breathing while asleep by providing a positive pressure in the throat. This small positive pressure prevents the airways collapsing during expiration. The CPAP machine takes some getting used to, and the noise generated by the device can also disturb the sleep of a bed partner. Therefore, many people (around half) do not use the device for long, or all night, and give up after three months.[30]

Supported Breathing

Many people with respiratory disease require breathing support, most often the breathing of supplementary oxygen supplied by a mask. The most common condition is COPD. Every year millions die from COPD, which is largely preventable as in most cases it is caused by breathing smoke from cigarettes, either tobacco or other substances such as marijuana, smoke from woodfires (used for cooking, for example), or fumes generated by gas cookers. Today tobacco-smoking is by far the greatest cause of COPD, which is a complex disease that develops slowly in smokers and usually appears in later life. Tobacco smoke, even filtered, contains many chemicals that over time irritate the lungs and cause irreversible damage. The smoker first notices that they are short of breath, have an expectorant cough in the morning, and catch more colds. If smoking continues, then the lungs become more obstructed, the symptoms get worse and breathing can become more laboured. Eventually supplemental oxygen is required and the smoker becomes breathless even when performing simple tasks such as getting dressed. The breathlessness associated with severe COPD is described as 'air hunger' and is particularly unpleasant. COPD sufferers will avoid the sensation as much as they can and become inactive as a result, which then leads to more disability. The condition is a complex one, hence its name: 'chronic' refers to the fact that it is a long-term condition, which in this case is irreversible. 'Obstructive' describes the fact that the airways become blocked and the lung architecture damaged, making breathing harder. 'Pulmonary' refers to reduced circulatory and cardiac function.

This modern description and name, COPD, has evolved by consensus from a gradual realization of its existence as a specific condition. The two main presenting symptoms are emphysema (from the Greek *emphusan*, 'to puff up'), where anatomical changes to the lung occur. The lung loses its fine spongey structure, which is destroyed and replaced by large, empty, gas-filled spaces. These spaces do not function well in gas exchange, so oxygen uptake and carbon dioxide exchange are reduced. The other recognizable symptom is chronic bronchitis, in which the lungs are inflamed and infected. The airways become blocked with excess mucus, which again limits gas exchange. At first these conditions were considered separate and treated as different diseases.

The earliest descriptions of emphysema were reported in 1679 by Théophile Bonet, a physician of Geneva who described 'voluminous' lungs, and by the Italian anatomist Giovanni Battista Morgagni in 1769 who reported nineteen cases of turgid, air-filled lungs.[31] It was the English physician Charles Badham whose 1814 book *An Essay on Bronchitis: With a Supplement Containing Remarks on Simple Pulmonary Abscess* was the first to define bronchitis as a separate condition. Thus a patient with emphysema and/or bronchitis could be treated differently from someone with asthma. A modern description of emphysema was given by the Frenchman René Laënnec, the inventor of the first monaural

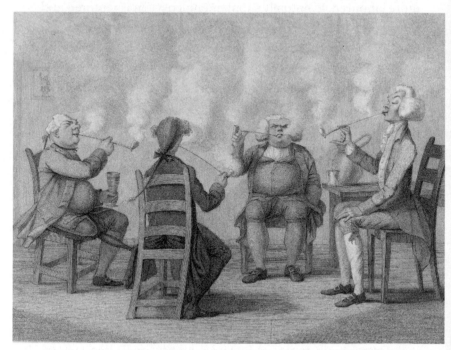

Stipple print by H. Bunbury, *c.* 1794. Four Georgian gentlemen at their club seriously engaged in smoking.

stethoscope. In his work of 1821, *A Treatise of Diseases of the Chest and on Mediate Auscultation*, he reported patients with both emphysema and chronic bronchitis (often called chronic catarrh). He died early at 45 years old of TB, a major hazard of treating patients with infectious chest diseases.

Before smoking was popularized during the First World War, COPD was rare and was either caused by a genetic predisposition or exposure to airborne pollutants of industrial origin, such as sulphur and nitrogen oxides and of course smoke. As such, many physicians ignored the condition, meaning it did not feature much in the medical literature. It was not until the 1950s that doctors began to notice an increased rate of emphysema and chronic bronchitis in tobacco smokers. Chronic sufferers exhibited a diversity of signs and symptoms depending on the proportions of emphysema or chronic bronchitis they suffered from, but all noticed that breathing had become more laboured.

Doctors noticed that patients broadly fell into two groups, which they termed 'pink puffers' and 'blue bloaters'. The pink puffers would be typically older and thin, with muscle wasting, and had unrelenting and disabling breathlessness and emphysema. Blue bloaters were often younger, overweight and with chronic bronchitis, leading to a purulent cough accompanied by heart failure. The two colours referred to the appearance of the skin. In blue bloaters, who are often overweight, the blueness or cyanosis resulted from the person having a low blood oxygen level (hypoxemia). The brain and regulatory systems readjust to tolerate a higher blood CO_2, and so do not fight to maintain normal blood gas levels. This saves energy, as the work of breathing is kept to a minimum. Patients breathe at a normal rate and are not breathless, but they are still low on oxygen.[32] Pink puffers are plethoric: that is, their skin is engorged with fine blood vessels, thus becoming pink. In these people the blood is well oxygenated, as the person over breathes (puffing) in order to remove excess blood carbon dioxide. Thus they seem to be fighting to breathe. Nowadays these terms are no longer used, as diagnosis and modern treatment methods have improved these symptoms.

Dying from end-stage COPD can result from type 1 or type 2 respiratory failure. Type 1 is due to a failure to oxygenate, where lung ventilation is inadequate; the person finds it difficult to breathe sufficiently to supply enough oxygen to the body. The extra work of breathing ultimately leads to the failure of the respiratory system and death. The initial stages of failure can be supported by supplementary oxygen, which increases the supply at the same ventilation rate. Type 2 respiratory failure results from inadequate ventilation also, but here the blood CO_2 is high and oxygen is low. Mechanical ventilation is used to treat severe respiratory failure.

Although the medical profession no longer refers to patients as pink puffers or blue bloaters, some speleologists (cavers) use the terms, particular in Australia. The caving fraternity do not use the terms medically but in a colloquial sense. Caves often contain 'foul air', not unlike mines. Depending on its geology and shape, a cave can contain elevated levels of carbon dioxide while still having normal oxygen levels, or a cave containing decomposing organic matter may have a reduced oxygen level or a significantly raised methane level. Cavers who enter these caves may respond in two ways: the majority respond by breathing faster, which makes their skin become pinker (if fair-skinned), the pink puffers. Those who are CO_2-tolerant do not increase their breathing rate and so can become cyanosed and faint: blue bloaters. Losing consciousness can be fatal if caving alone.

Many tobacco smokers do not suffer any ill effects from smoking whatsoever, but a sizable proportion do, and these may include not only COPD but cardiovascular disease and cancer. Apart from nicotine, tobacco smoke contains thousands of compounds, around 250 of which can cause mouth, throat, bladder and lung cancer. Indeed, it was the rapid rise in lung cancer in the last century that alerted doctors to the toxicity of breathing tobacco smoke. Lung cancer was extremely rare before the twentieth century and was often misdiagnosed as TB or pneumonia.[33] Later the increase in lung cancer was blamed on poison gas exposure during the First World War, on the great influenza pandemic of 1918–20 and later on the tar used in the making of many new tarmac roads.

The first hint that smoking was unhealthy came in the 1930s, when the first clinical trials were conducted. It was noted that the lung cancer group contained more smokers than the lung-cancer-free group. After the Second World War, research resumed, resulting in the 1950s in two large studies, one in the UK (comparing smoking and non-smoking doctors) and one in the USA, a study of 187,766 men. The authors of these studies stated that the link between smoking tobacco and lung cancer had been proven 'beyond a reasonable doubt'.[34] Along with confirmatory results from animal studies, the results shocked the public, who had been told that smoking was harmless and even healthy. As a result confidence in smoking and smoking rates collapsed. The world's tobacco manufacturers did not issue a health warning about their products, but instead decided to counter the evidence and refute the findings in the scientific and clinical press and to actively generate general public ignorance of this link.[35] With their vast financial reserves they conducted successful campaigns, which from the 1950s onwards led to increased smoking rates, which peaked in the 1980s.

After this, the tide began to turn, as public health bodies in the wealthier countries of Europe and North America launched equally effective counter-advertising campaigns. With government help smoking was heavily taxed and followed in many countries by bans on smoking in public places. Smoking was further reduced by the invention of nicotine patches and electronic cigarettes and vaping, which uses nebulized nicotine mist. In the UK smoking rates have dropped from around 60 per cent of men and 40 per cent of women in the 1950s to around 15 per cent of the population in 2019. Though smoking rates have continued to drop in Europe and North America, it has risen in Asia, particularly in China and India. In China, where the government manufactures the cigarettes, it quadrupled between 1980 and 2010, with 2,000 billion cigarettes smoked per year. While about 100 million people died from smoking-related disease in the twentieth century, the

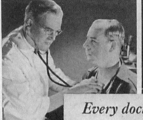
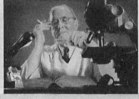
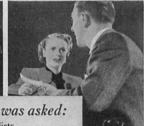
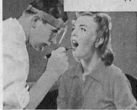
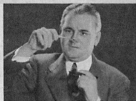
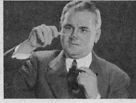

Cigarette advert from the late 1940s, directed at both doctors and the general public, which subtly sought to subvert emerging statistical and epidemiological evidence by inviting doctors and patients to 'make your own test'.

number in the twenty-first century is predicted to be much larger, as it takes around 25 years of smoking before symptoms appear. The intensity and dishonesty of tobacco industry advertising campaigns have had the greatest impact on the history of breathing. We were told that smoking improved respiratory health, and then, as the evidence began to show otherwise, smoking was depicted in a positive social light. The notion of brand loyalty was ruthlessly exploited by the advertising industry, and as all smokers were addicted to nicotine there was a guaranteed pool of customers. It was two decades, the 1950s and '60s, before breathlessness, ill health and the early symptoms of COPD and lung cancer began to appear in large numbers. Today we are exposed to similar advertising messages from the fast-food industry, which deliberately tries to generate ignorance about the link of its products to obesity.

Respiratory disease accounts for 1 in 5 deaths in the world and 1 in 8 deaths in Europe, around 600,000 per year. Half of these deaths are due to lung cancer or COPD linked to smoking. Many smokers begin in their youth, when they are totally unaware of the ways that impaired breathing can disable the body and cause grave illness, such as cancer. These are seen as diseases of old age. By the time smokers are middle-aged they are addicted to tobacco.[36]

THE CESSATION OF breathing for more a few minutes leads ultimately to death. This can result from nervous diseases, with faults focused centrally in the brain, or peripherally in the thorax, with the nerves signalling muscle contraction. Alternatively, it can result from injury or trauma. We risk death if our lungs are filled with water or we are crushed by an overwhelming force. The ability to restore breathing has taken many centuries of effort, some of which has occurred through serendipity or via the concentrated work of physicians, engineers and scientists. Often under conditions of great adversity, we have overcome the problems of exposing the lungs to excess negative or positive pressure, and invented mechanical devices that can support breathing for many months or even years. Finally, we have developed face masks that, when worn while asleep or during the day, can aid breathing by splinting open the airways with pressure or enhance blood oxygen levels by supplying oxygen-enriched air to breathe. Our perception of breathing has been altered by the global phenomenon of smoking, which has given a close-up view of how valuable it is to breathe clean air.

SIX

BREATHING HIGH AND LOW

B reathing changes with exertion and stress, both physical and emotional. In team sports such as football or individual sports such as marathon running, all participants become breathless, either in short bursts or throughout the duration of the sporting event. Increased performance and fitness necessitate breathing faster and deeper. Some recreational activities such as swimming and rowing place even greater demands on breathing, as performance and breathing rate are intertwined. For other sports, such as archery, breathing gets in the way, so holding the breath is required. Living or exercising at high altitude alters breathing, as at higher altitudes oxygen availability lessens: the atmosphere thins the higher that one is above sea level. Conversely, the atmospheric pressure increases when we drop below sea level, during diving, for instance. Under these extreme circumstances, breathing and the respiratory system respond in a variety of diverse ways.

There are also many occasions when we consciously alter our breathing: to play instruments such as the trumpet and flute, to sing, to ululate and speak. Our unconscious self has a profound impact on our breathing; our emotions can dictate our long-term breathing or hijack it for a brief period. As we experience joy, we laugh; sadness, we cry; and boredom, we yawn.

Breathing Hard

During short bursts of exertion, such as rushing to catch a train before it pulls off from the platform or while sprinting 100 metres, breathing tends to be secondary. The mind is usually more focused on the immediate task ahead. We stop to notice our breathing only once the exertion is over, when we pant, breathe rapidly, sweat a little and relax. This breathless feeling or air hunger is not considered a sign of ill health but a normal response. While not associated with lung disease, the duration, unpleasantness or intensity of this breathlessness is augmented by increased age, smoking, being overweight and sometimes being in a heightened emotional state.

Running, one of the commonest forms of exercise, can be done in short bursts lasting a few seconds or a marathon lasting hours. Our breathing rate has to be very adaptable to respond to these different situations. The current world record for running 100 metres is 9.572 seconds, set by the Jamaican Usain Bolt in 2009, and an amazing 8.7 seconds (around 42 kph) with a running start. For female athletes, the corresponding record is 10.49 seconds, set by Florence Griffith-Joyner for the USA in 1988. Given that the average breath takes around 3–4 seconds to complete, there is little time to breathe during the 100 metres. In this race the huge amount of energy expended needs to be obtained from the oxygen already in the blood, with the majority of the required energy coming from the chemical energy already stored in the muscles (so-called anaerobic, 'without oxygen', metabolism). The aerobic system (metabolism that relies on oxygen) contributes around 10 per cent in males during this event.[1] The contribution of the aerobic system increases as the duration of exercise increases, so during the 400 metres the contribution is around 40 per cent and in the 800 metres 60 per cent in males and 70 per cent in women.[2] The official fastest times for these two distances are 43.03 and 47.06 seconds (set by Wayde van Niekerk from South Africa and Marita Koch from Germany) and 100.91 and 113.28 seconds (set by David Rudisha from Kenya, and Jarmila Kratochvílová from

Czechoslovakia, now Czechia), respectively. Roughly speaking, bouts of exercise lasting less than 75 seconds are fuelled without extra oxygen.[3] The effects of this acute oxygen lack are felt after exertion. When you run for a train about to leave the platform, if you are lucky enough to board, you spend the first minute or two breathing rapidly, 'catching your breath' and feeling warm. Although no longer exercising, you breathe deeply and rapidly as if you are. The body is responding to an oxygen debt. Breathing settles down only once the blood oxygen levels return to pre-exertion levels and in parallel have expelled all the excess carbon dioxide generated by burning glucose. This oxygen debt is even more obvious in athletes who, after completing the 100-metre race, dramatically collapse onto the track, often lying prostrate for some considerable time, grimacing with exhaustion. Only the victors ignore this painful debt to oxygen, staying on their feet to acknowledge the cheers and applause of their audience.

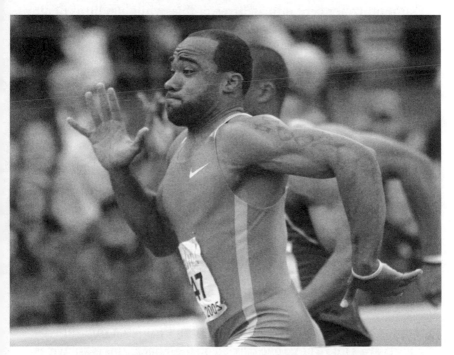

Anwar Moore running the 100 metres at the annual Spitzen Leichathletic track and field event in June 2005, here with his mouth closed. Over such a short distance, breathing adds little to performance.

In longer races or bouts of exercise, oxygen uptake and carbon dioxide generation and excretion are important and limit performance. The two processes are determined by how quickly gas exchange occurs in the lungs and tissues. With long bouts of exertion, it is not possible to live off an oxygen debt, so the lungs and heart have no alternative but to perform more efficiently. While humans exercise, the breathing rate and heart rate can only increase three- to fourfold above resting. The amount the lungs can inhale during a single breath can increase around sevenfold while the quantity of blood the heart can pump each beat can increase around threefold. This allows the maximum quantity of air that can be inhaled during exercise to increase from around 7 litres per minute to 180 litres a minute, a 26-fold increase, and likewise the amount of blood being pumped around the body from 5 to 35 litres per minute, a sevenfold increase. At rest 7 litres of air contains around 1.5 litres of oxygen, and the body uses only around 17 per cent or 0.25 litres of this, while 180 litres of air contain 38 litres of oxygen. An exercising man of average build would consume around 2.8 litres or 7 per cent of this at his most active. For an elite athlete the numbers would be a lot more impressive. Disturbed oxygen levels are not the only thing that change breathing: the extra carbon dioxide will also increase the stimulus to breathe, as will the associated increase in blood acid load.

In 1922 the British physiologist Archibald Vivian Hill coined the terms 'maximal oxygen consumption' and 'oxygen debt', the same year he received his Nobel Prize in Physiology and Medicine.[4] The Nobel Prize was for his work elucidating the mechanism of heat production in working muscles. Hill was a keen runner, and more than likely a subject in his papers, as the age given for one of his study participants matches Hill's age of 35. In the study the subject runs around an open-air track (of 92½-yard or 84.6-metre circumference) while breathing through a mouthpiece and valves into a large bag carried on their back. This is known as a Douglas bag, and has greatly contributed to our understanding of breathing.

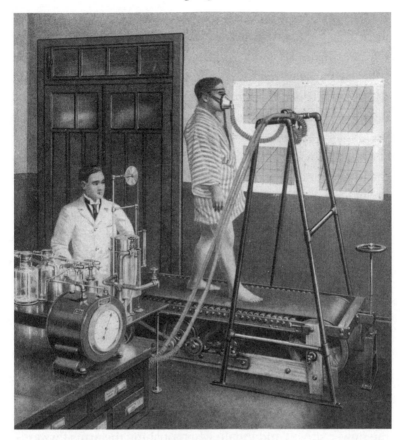

Halftone illustration (1929–30) documenting the investigation of respiration during exercise. While the subject exercises on a primitive treadmill he breathes into a mask and exhalations are measured by a gas metre on the nearby bench, which includes a spirometer. Today the scientific equipment has been miniaturized and the subject's safety is paramount.

The science behind the Douglas bag is simple. The idea is that if you could capture each expired breath, you could then measure its size and composition and thus work out the body's rate of oxygen use (inspired air has a known composition) and calorics. (The inventor Claude Gordon Douglas (1882–1963) was a contemporary of Haldane and worked at the University of Oxford. He was one of the experts who worked on the chemical gas attacks of the First World War.) The original bag was wedge-shaped, made of twill cloth and lined with vulcanized rubber, and held 50 litres of gas when full.[5] The rubberized layer and valves prevented the expired gas from leaking away or changing composition. By collecting expiration, the total volume of gas expelled, amount of oxygen consumed and carbon dioxide produced over a certain time can easily be determined in the laboratory later. Although gas bags had been used for decades before Douglas's, none had been gas-proof. The simple Douglas bag and the ability to measure metabolism and gas exchange revolutionized sport and exercise science for the next fifty or more years, as well as contributing to the understanding of aviation and diving physiology. Nowadays the Douglas bag has been superseded by electronic gas and flow analysers that are small enough to be worn by the athlete and measure oxygen consumption many times a second, allowing breath-by-breath calculation of metabolism.

In some sports deeper and faster breathing is not the only issue. Rowing and swimming require cyclical manoeuvres of the upper body. Matching each stroke of the oar or arm with exhalation improves performance greatly. When swimming the body is in a horizontal position and immersed in water, a much denser medium than air, so a swimmer has to work harder to breathe. Entrainment of arm strokes with breathing helps reduce this work. Most swimmers exhale when pulling their arms backwards (called the power stroke) and inhale when pushing the arms forwards, ready for the next stroke. Rowing presents different challenges. It can place a lot of stress on the breathing muscles of the chest, so matching breathing rhythm to the rowing rate helps to reduce this stress and so improves the efficiency of rowing. Rowers are encouraged to breathe through their mouths. When rowing at a slow pace, exhalation is taken when the oars are pulled back for the power stroke, with exhalation finishing when the hands reach the body. Inhalation occurs during recovery when the oars are lifted from the water and pushed forward. Consciously forcing the exhalation in time with each stroke requires considerable training, more so than the actual act of rowing itself. With a much faster rowing rate, breathing becomes more complicated, and two breaths are required per stroke, with a quick exhalation added when recovering the oars for the next stroke. This entrainment of breathing rate and rowing frequency allows rowing coordination while at the same time supporting muscle aerobic respiration. We are all well used to adapting our breathing rhythm, as we do this all the time when we eat and swallow food or drink liquid. To ensure that food enters the oesophagus instead of the trachea, we need to coordinate our breathing and swallowing, for without it food and liquid would enter the lungs.

As Galen observed, breathing is paced by a small island of tissue in the brain stem. This nerve centre interprets and integrates all the signals arriving from around the body, and moment by moment generates a respiratory rhythm and pattern, which drives the lungs to contract and relax, leading to an appropriate breathing rate. Unconsciously, through feedback from stretch receptors in the lungs and chemoreceptors in the arteries and brain, the respiratory centre is influenced by exercise, body cooling, heating, hypoxia (lack of oxygen), pain and panic, which often increase the breathing rate.[6] These changes can occur without any conscious perception. We remain unaware of them until respiratory discomfort occurs and a behavioural system in the higher brain is switched on. Upon becoming aware, our perception of breathlessness motivates avoidance behaviour such as reducing activity, seeking fresh air by opening the window, distracting ourselves, using an inhaler spray or even seeking medical help. The linking of physiological and behavioural sensing, so-called interoception, allows us to respond appropriately to our current environment.[7] People describe breathlessness in various ways, as either having to breathe too much or not being able to breathe enough. Others describe a need to take deep breaths or gasps, a feeling of suffocation or a tightness in the chest (as if a tight band is around it) or throat.[8] Emotions alter our breathing rate and slowing our breathing rate via meditation leads to a feeling of well-being. Negative emotions such as anger and fear have the opposite effect, increasing the breathing rate. This is an appropriate response and subsides once the emotion subsides.

However, the breathing response to an emotional disturbance can be inappropriate. One such condition is called a panic attack.

Such an attack can be triggered by fears, such as agoraphobia, or by particular situations. Sometimes they happen without any obvious cause. During a panic attack, our inbuilt defensive response to stress is inappropriately triggered.[9] The mechanism of panic attacks is not fully known, but evidence suggests that breathing fast, or hyperventilating, is triggered by raised carbon dioxide levels, or in some cases obstructed breathing. What is known is that there are psychological components to the attack, with a panic threesome – interoception, conditioning and fear – working together.[10] This disorder can be treated by avoiding the trigger(s), and engaging in deconditioning processes and cognitive behavioural therapy.

This link between breathing, body, motor control (movement and postural position) and cognitive awareness can be best demonstrated when playing music. One Japanese study of pianists showed that breathing changed depending on the piece of classical music played, be it Mozart or Debussy, and also between individual musicians.[11]

Breathing at High Altitude

Most world and Olympic athletics records are achieved in big city venues, usually when a large audience is present. Most of these venues are at low altitudes, at most a few hundred metres above sea level. One exception was the 1968 Summer Olympics in Mexico City, around 2,250 metres (7,400 ft) above sea level. The atmosphere thins with increasing altitude. The composition stays the same – sea level air is composed of 21 per cent oxygen, just as it is on top of Mount Everest at 8,848 metres (29,029 ft) – but what is different is the air pressure. At sea level the atmospheric pressure is typically 760 mmHg, or 1 atmosphere, while on top of Everest it is around 250 mmHg, a third of what most of us are used to. The consequence of this low barometric pressure is that the ratio of external to internal oxygen pressure is lower, which can lead to poor oxygen uptake and tissue hypoxia. Thus people who climb Everest require oxygen support, especially if they hope to reach the summit. Some climbers have made it to the summit without extra oxygen and survived, while others have died because they spent too long on the summit and ran out of supplementary oxygen. At sea level this reduced pressure would be equivalent to an atmosphere containing around 6 per cent oxygen and would require a supplement of around 75 per cent oxygen to bring it up to the normal levels we experience.

At altitude, the lower oxygen pressure in the blood at first raises the breathing rate, which is good at increasing blood oxygen, but as this hyperventilation reduces the blood carbon dioxide content, breathing eventually slows. This slowing then worsens the hypoxia. With time, usually after a week, the body acclimatizes to these conditions and any ill effects, such as dizziness or fainting, disappear. If the changes in ambient air pressure are too quick, then the person can black out, something that happens when pilots fly too high.

Apart from acclimatization, other altitude-related conditions occur. Acute mountain sickness (AMS) can occur above 2,500 metres (8,200 ft) and tends to become more severe above 3,600 metres (12,000 ft). It is characterized by headache, nausea, fatigue, anorexia (loss of appetite), breathlessness and difficulty in sleeping.[12] The severity varies from mild and inconvenient to severe and life-threatening. It becomes so when there is fluid build-up (oedema) in either the brain or lungs, or both. Slowing the rate of ascent to altitude reduces the chances of getting symptoms. Around half of mountaineers experience AMS to some extent, while in tourists who visit or stay at mountain resorts it is around a quarter. When climbing higher than 3,000 metres (10,000 ft), a small number of mountaineers develop the more serious condition of high-altitude cerebral oedema (HACO or HACE, following the American spelling of 'edema'), in which the brain swells with fluid, or high-altitude pulmonary oedema (HAPO or HAPE), in which fluid builds up in the lungs instead. Sleeping at high altitude can contribute to these conditions, as during sleep breathing patterns are altered and frequent apnoeas (short periods when breathing stops) can occur, leading to hypoxia and poor sleep.

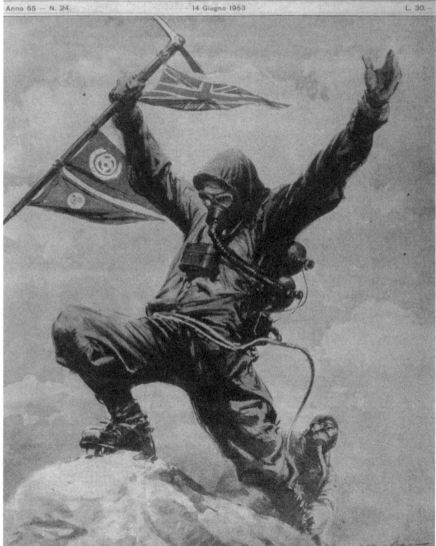

LA DOMENICA DEL CORRIERE

Supplemento settimanale illustrato del nuovo CORRIERE DELLA SERA - Abbonamenti: Italia, anno L. 1400, sem. L. 750 - Estero, anno L. 2000, sem. L. 1050

Anno 55 — N. 24   14 Giugno 1953   L. 30.—

Conquistata la vetta del mondo. Una cordata della spedizione britannica, composta dal neozelandese Hillary e dalla guida nepalese Tensing, ha raggiunto, con l'aiuto di apparecchi respiratori ad ossigeno, la vetta dell'Everest (m. 8888) la massima elevazione della Terra, che aveva finora respinto dieci tentativi. Sulla cima sono state spiegate al vento tre piccole bandiere: della Gran Bretagna, delle Nazioni Unite e del Nepal. (Disegno di Walter Molino)

New Zealand's Edmund Hillary and Nepalese Sherpa Tenzing Norgay are the first to reach the summit of Mount Everest (at 8,848 m) in May 1953, both wearing 'open-circuit' oxygen breathing apparatus and carrying oxygen cylinders on their backs. Cover of *La Domenica del Corriere*, 14 June 1953.

Supplying oxygen or returning to lower altitudes usually resolves most of the symptoms, which are reversible, although some people complain of long-term impairment of vision.

Long-term exposure to high altitude is very limited in Europe, with its highest Alpine mountain being Mount Blanc, France, at 4,810 metres (15,780 ft). The highest towns in Europe are located at around 1,000 metres (mostly in the Pyrenees mountains, where the winter weather is not so severe as in the Alps). Alpine meadows are open to grazing and farming in the summer months but are inhospitable in the colder winter. Although they form a natural geographical barrier and are an environmental challenge in the winter, we know that the Alps were populated all year around from archaeological finds dating back to the Neolithic. Even the higher portions were populated, as the discovery of the 5,000-year-old Ice or Similaun Man 3,210 metres (10,530 ft) up the Ötzal Alps in 1991 proves. No special physiological adaptation is needed to live at the altitude of the lower slopes (typically below 1,000 metres, or 3,300 ft). Most Europeans were adapted to living at sea level. This changed when in the 1500s the Spanish travelled to South America, where in the Andes they came across indigenous populations living at extreme altitudes above 2,500 metres (8,200 ft).

By the sixteenth century the Spanish in South America had slowly overcome the Inca Empire and by 1533 the Inca capital Cusco was under Spanish administration. The Inca Empire was in the western range of the Andes, covering Peru, Chile and Ecuador. Although Cusco is situated in a basin of a fertile valley, it sits at an altitude of around 3,400 metres (11,200 ft). The indigenous population at this time was around 200,000 and were acclimatized to living at this altitude. The Spanish on the contrary found the altitude uncomfortable and complained that the air was much too thin, leaving them feeling breathless. Thus, over forty years, the Spanish relocated the capital to Lima on the coast, which is now the capital of Peru, with a population of more than 10 million in 2020. Cusco with a population of around 500,000 in 2017, is now a popular place for visitors as it contains many archaeological remains of the Inca Empire. Even today foreign visitors who fly into Lima are advised not to visit Cusco directly but to travel there over a few days, increasing the altitude slowly so as to allow time for acclimatization. Alternatively, many people with less time on their hands instead visit Machu Picchu, 80 kilometres (50 mi.) north of Cusco. The ruin is located in a spectacular location in the mountains but at a much lower altitude of 2,430 metres (7,090 ft) above sea level, so is less likely to cause altitude sickness when visited just for the day.

Around the world there are several regions where people live at high altitudes (above 2,500 metres). There are three Andean Altiplanos in South America, the Tibetan plateau in Asia and the Semien Plateau in Ethiopia. Today around 150 million people live at high altitude. These indigenous populations show physiological adaption to the low oxygen levels. These adaptions have evolved over many generations and via genetic selection. The three geographical populations have differing solutions to the problem of reduced oxygen availability. The other factor, cold temperatures, plays only a small role.

The indigenous Andean population who have lived at high altitudes for many thousands of years have physiologically adapted to altitude by having a higher blood haemoglobin concentration, with typically 3 to 4 grams more per litre of blood than their fellow-countrymen who live at lower altitude.[13] Having more of the oxygen-carrying protein allows them to carry more oxygen in their blood per litre than lowlanders. This is the rationale behind training at altitude, increasing the haemoglobin concentration naturally and not by doping. Having a high blood haemoglobin concentration has its risks though, as the blood is more viscous, which places a greater strain on the heart. Christina Eichstaedt and her colleagues from the UK compared two Andean populations, the Calchaquíes, who reside at 2,500 metres (8,200 ft) and the Collas, who live at 3,500 metres (11,482 ft), with one living at sea level, the Wichí. They found major differences between the three groups, showing as expected that those at the highest altitudes had the most obvious adaptions to their oxygen carry capacity and mechanical lung function, and at rest breathed more rapidly than their sea-level counterparts, at 21 compared to 18 breaths per minute. This is a small but significant difference, especially when this represents a lifetime of extra work for the respiratory muscles. The intermediate population were less distinctive and exhibited a mixture of adaptations, for instance not breathing more rapidly, but still being lighter than the lowlanders, as were the Collas.

Today, La Paz, Bolivia, is the highest capital city in the world; with a population close to a million, it sits at around 3,600 metres (11,811 ft). The average person who flies into La Paz feels some form of breathlessness, while the local population walk around as if at sea level.

The Tibetan population show a completely different adaptation to altitude. While they exhibit normal or reduced blood haemoglobin levels, they instead breathe more rapidly, exhibiting a respiratory response to hypoxia. Recent scientists have shown that the indigenous Tibetans (the Sherpa) inherited these qualities, traits and characteristics many thousands of years ago.[14] The indigenous Tibetan DNA contains sequences from extinct or archaic humans, the hominins Neanderthals and Denisovans. Neanderthal bones have been found across Europe, the Near East and Central Asia, allowing their DNA to be sequenced. Denisovan finds are much rarer, with the first discoveries of a few bones and teeth unearthed in the frozen Denisova Cave in the Siberian Altai mountains in 2010. The cave was also occupied by Neanderthals and modern humans in turn. The remains were from a teenage girl who died over 90,000 years ago. DNA extracted from her bones showed that her mother was Neanderthal and father Denisovan. Another find was of a 160,000-year-old jaw, this time in Baishiya Karst Cave on the Tibetan plateau, Xiahe, Gansu, China.[15] The cave is at an altitude of 3,280 metres (10,761 ft), showing that these hominins adapted to living at altitude well before the arrival of *Homo sapiens*. How they breathed at these hypoxic altitudes has yet to be discovered. There is proof that the Denisovans survived until modern times and interbred with modern humans, as both

Neanderthal and Denisovan DNA is present in our modern human genome and found in many people, such as Melanesians and Aboriginals. In the Tibetan population about 0.4 per cent of the genome is introgressed (integrated) with Denisovan DNA, providing the genetic legacy that allows the Tibetans to tolerate high-altitude living.

People living in the Ethiopian highlands live at around 3,000 metres (9,800 ft). The indigenous population has adapted to living at altitude in a similar manner to the Andeans by increasing their blood haemoglobin concentration. Their blood oxygen carriage is less efficient than the blood found in their Andean counterparts.

In Europe the acute effects of altitude on breathing were quickly discovered after the invention of the hot air balloon. Unlike climbing a mountain (before the invention of cable cars), hot air balloons could ascend very quickly to heights unimaginable before the eighteenth century. Balloons big enough to carry humans skyward began with the French Montgolfier brothers, Joseph-Michel (1740–1810) and Jacques-Étienne (1745–1799). It seems bizarre to us today that they believed that it was the smoke generated by fires that provided lift (like a cloud), not hot air, so their cloth and paper balloons were filled using bonfires built with smoke-generating materials such as straw and old shoes. These were called fire balloons; it was only later that the term 'hot air balloon' was coined, when it was realized that it was the less dense heated air that lifted the balloon, not the smoke. The brothers' first public unmanned ascent was in June 1783, and a great success. This stimulated another sibling pair, the Robert brothers, Anne-Jean (1758–1820) and Nicolas-Louis (1760–1820), to become balloon builders. The pair took a more sophisticated approach, producing a rubberized balloon that allowed them to use hydrogen gas as a lifting agent. Their first public unmanned launch was in August 1783, inflated with 34,000 litres of hydrogen, allowing the balloon to stay airborne indefinitely. By the autumn, on 19 September, the Montgolfiers conducted their first 'manned' flight by adding a basket containing a sheep, rooster and a duck.[16]

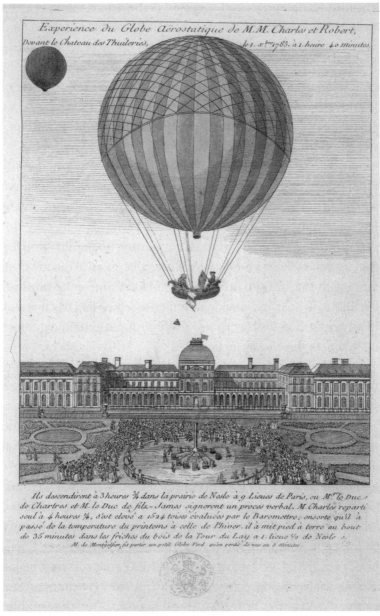

Engraving (1780–1810) documenting the first ascent in a hydrogen gas filled balloon, in 1783, by Jacques Charles and Anne-Jean Robert. Beginning from the Tuileries Palace, the flight lasted one hour and forty minutes, ending up 44 kilometres (27 mi.) away in the town of Nesle.

The next obvious prize was manned flight, and it was suggested by the king, Louis XVI, that the animals be replaced by two convicts, rather than risking the Montgolfiers themselves. Instead, in November, with the view to becoming the world's first aeronauts, Jean François Pilâtre de Rozier, a physicist and then Director of the Royal Museum, and a friend ascended to 900 metres (2,950 ft), staying aloft for 20 minutes and covering 8 kilometres (5 mi.) while suffering no ill effects.[17]

Two years later, in 1785, Pilâtre de Rozier was killed while attempting to balloon across the English Channel. His fire-balloon caught fire at 914 metres (3,000 ft) and crashed to the ground. A few weeks later the Robert brothers took to the air in their hydrogen balloon. Watched by a crowd containing Benjamin Franklin, they stayed aloft for 2 hours, travelling 32 kilometres (20 mi.) and landing as the sun set. Excited by the flight, one of the brothers decided to fly solo and quickly ascended to 10,000 ft (3,048 metres), nearly rupturing his eardrums. This painful experience put him off taking to the air any further.[18]

Within fifty or sixty years balloon aeronauts were travelling hundreds of kilometres, for example in the USA flying the 1,800 kilometres (1,120 mi.) from St Louis to New York. Most of these early flights were at relatively low altitude not surpassing 6,000 metres (20,000 ft), although some aeronauts commented that at this altitude breathing rate increased along with heart rate and some people exhibited purple faces. It was the first scientific flights that were to provide new insights to breathing in rarefied air. In September 1865 two Englishmen, Henry Coxwell and James Glaisher, in a balloon filled with the newly invented coal gas, briefly reached 11,887 metres (39,000 ft) and barely survived, losing consciousness owing to the low oxygen pressure (144 mmHg) and extreme cold (-11°C, or 12.2°F). It was soon realized that supplemental oxygen was needed to go higher and to remain at these altitudes for longer periods. In 1875, a French crew, Theodore Sivel, Joseph Croce-Spinelli and Gaston Tissandier, in a balloon called the *Zenith*, set out to beat the altitude record by taking bags of air enriched with oxygen with them. The flight was scientifically planned by Paul Bert, who realized after the launch that the aeronauts did not have enough oxygen. They started inhaling the oxygen at 7,010 metres (23,000 ft) but began to suffer from the cold. Suffering from hypothermia, they were barely able to breathe the bagged oxygen, and all passed out as the balloon continued to ascend rapidly. The balloon reached 8,534 metres (28,000 ft) before descending on its own. At around 3,048 metres (10,000 ft) Tissandier awoke and managed to land the balloon safely. The other two were dead, and frozen stiff. These were the first deaths on a scientific ballooning expedition. Paul Bert in their eulogy stated:

> They ascend and death seizes them, without a struggle, without suffering, as a prey fallen to it on those icy regions where an eternal silence reigns. Yes, our unhappy friends have had this strange privilege, this fatal honour, of being the first to die in the heavens.[19]

These weren't the last deaths in the air. In 1927 Captain Hawthorne C. Gray of the u.s. Army Corps died of hypoxia after reaching a record altitude of 13,220 metres (43,380 ft) in a helium balloon. The current altitude record was set in 2014, when Alan Eustace reached 41,420 metres (135,906 ft) in a helium balloon with a pressurized gondola below. The highest hot air balloon ascent was set in 2005, made by Vijaypat Singhania to 21,290 metres (69,850 ft).

With the invention of the aeroplane, pilots soon matched the altitudes reached by balloonists, Guido Guidi reaching 7,900 metres (26,083 ft) in 1916. By the Second World War the altitude record was 17,330 metres (56,850 ft), set by Lt Colonel Mario Prezzi of the Italian Air Force, wearing a pressure suit.

Before the Second World War flying was a privilege, with a few small airline services carrying passengers here and there. During the war the RAF had grown enormously, with over a million personnel by 1944, while the United States Army Air Forces had 2.5 million personnel. Not all of these people were aircrew, but a good proportion flew in the hundreds of thousands of planes and missions. The pilots who flew these unpressurized planes were often overcome by hypoxia, leading to confusion and disorientation, even at 3,000 metres. After the war oxygen masks were used, and the altitude record grew and grew until it reached the edge of the atmosphere, the so-called Kármán line, at 100,000 metres (330,000 ft or 62 miles). The line was named after Theodore von Kármán (1881–1963), an engineer and physicist who calculated the height of this boundary.

Heavy Breathing

Breathing above sea level becomes laboured as the air becomes thinner, so the opposite should be the case below sea level as the air becomes heavier. On Earth this is not something we notice, as most of its low-lying surfaces are submerged below the sea or the ice floes of Antarctica. There are a few low-lying areas, such as the dry Death Valley in California which is 86 metres (282 ft) below sea level. Another area is around the Dead Sea, a salt lake situated between Jordan and Israel, which is one of the lowest places in the world. The lake shoreline is 413 metres (1,355 ft) below global sea level. The atmospheric pressure should on average be 5 per cent higher (21mm Hg) than the surrounding areas, which should have the positive effect of aiding the passage of oxygen into the blood. These advantages were recognized in 1876 by the British explorer Captain Sir Richard Francis Burton, who was famous for his clandestine travels around Asia, the Middle East and Africa. He stated:

> I proposed to utilize the regions around the Dead Sea . . . where oxygen accumulates and where, run as hard as you like, you can never be out of breath. This will be the great Consumptive hospital of the future.[20]

In a more recent study, it was found that people with COPD who underwent pulmonary rehabilitation at the Dead Sea were less breathless compared to those treated in nearby Jerusalem.[21] One recently discovered depression is a canyon in Antarctica that is 3,500 metres (11,400 ft) deep and around 62 km long. Being covered by the Denman Glacier, it is full of ice, but if it were accessible the air would be enriched with a 45 per cent increased oxygen pressure. The deepest accessible places are caves and mines. The deepest mines are the gold mines of South Africa, which can be 3,800 metres (12,467 ft) deep. Here the increased atmospheric and oxygen pressure are not an advantage to breathing. As in most deep mines, receiving adequate ventilation is a problem, and excessive carbon dioxide and carbon monoxide levels can quickly become hazardous.

Raised atmospheric pressure does alter breathing, but how we discovered this did not come from observing miners or residents of the Dead Sea, but from civil engineers. Before the eighteenth century, bridges were built largely of stone or wood. The largest bridges consisted of several stone arches standing in the water and were constructed to be strong enough to withstand the greatest flows following torrential rain. In the UK and Europe, the Industrial Revolution led to the building of the first substantial cast iron bridge in 1781, over the River Severn. Once iron and, later, steel were used in construction, larger spans became possible, and bridges could then traverse gorges and rivers without submerging arches in the water. Construction on the Clifton Suspension Bridge, spanning the Avon Gorge in Bristol and designed by Isambard Kingdom Brunel, started in 1831. It opened in 1864, with a final span of 214 metres (702 ft) and a length of 412 metres (1,352 ft). As civil engineers became more confident, the bridges got bigger. In the USA in the mid-nineteenth century, St Louis had become the gateway to the west. Here goods crossing from one U.S. coast to the other had to cross the Mississippi River by ferry, a hazardous manoeuvre during adverse winter weather. A bridge big enough to cross the river would have to stretch 460 metres (1,500 ft), making it the biggest in the world, and it wasn't until after the Civil War in 1864 that the plans to build a bridge began. The challenge was not the span itself but building the stone supports, as the river would be bridged with four piers and three spans. Two of the piers would need to be built midstream. In all the bridge would weigh 18,000 tonnes and require substantial supports. At the bridge site the bedrock was 27–34 metres (90–110 ft) below the river surface.

To dig down below the river bottom, watertight open-ended compartments called caissons would have to be sunk down to the river bottom. To prevent water leaking into the chamber, it would need to be constantly pressurized using compressed air. This allowed the workers to remove the riverbed in dry, safe conditions. This technology had been developed first in France in 1869 and used to dig a shaft 23 metres (75 ft) deep. When dropping a shaft underwater, the caisson air pressure increases by one atmosphere every 9 metres (30 ft) or so descended, so the French labourers had to work at over two atmospheres. With the St Louis bridge, four to five atmospheres of pressure were needed at the greatest depth. During construction, the bridge workers would work all day in these sealed caissons, leaving and entering through an airlock chamber. When entering the chamber, the airlock would be closed, and compressed air instantly fed into the room. This often caused earache and congestion (blocked nose and fluid retention), which would pass quickly. At the end of their shift, the opposite occurred, and once locked in the air lock chamber the atmospheric pressure was restored rapidly by opening the valves to let the compressed air flood out uncontrolled. This immediate decompression caused pain in the knee and elbow joints, so the workers typically waited 10 minutes before they left the depths of the caisson by climbing the stairs to the surface. The original French workers, after a few weeks of working, had developed a stooped walk, a condition which became known as the 'bends', and became the butt of jokes. When building the St Louis bridge the compression and decompression procedures did not change, despite the depth of the bed rock being deeper and therefore requiring greater air compression. In the American workers the bends were seen when they had excavated to a depth of 18 metres (60 ft), when the caisson pressure required to stop the surrounding water leaking in needed to be over two atmospheres. As the workers went deeper the effects of decompression became worse. On returning to the surface the joint pain was accompanied by muscle aches, headaches, dizziness (called the staggers), itching (the niggles) and shortness of breath (the chokes). The chokes are nowadays called pulmonary decompression sickness. The deeper they excavated, the worse the symptoms, and in addition came nausea, vomiting, and bleeding from the gums and ears. The first death occurred when they reached a depth of over 24 metres (90 ft) and were exposed to over three atmospheres of pressure. It occurred in a young healthy worker who, after climbing the stairs to the surface, started gasping for air before momentarily staggering and dying. A further six men died this way before the engineers decided to change the compression and decompression rates, transitioning from immediate decompression to a slower rate and allowing the air-lock pressure to equalize over 20 minutes. This prevented further deaths from the bends.

At the time, no one knew what caused Caisson disease (as it became known), and a number of theories were put forward. Some postulated that it was the simple effect of compression causing blood to engorge the internal organs and moving away from the periphery. This would account for the feelings of congestion. Other theories put the symptoms down to a raised carbon dioxide level in the caisson, as in this confined space there was plenty of manual labour and candles were used for illumination. The physician employed by the bridge builders, Antoine Alphonse Jaminet, who investigated the workers' symptoms, thought it was due to the movement of 'vital energy', which was somehow enhanced during compression and lost during decompression.

The French physician Paul Bert correctly identified nitrogen in the air as the problem. The air we breathe contains around 78 per cent nitrogen, which dissolves into the blood and tissues in proportion to its pressure. Unlike oxygen it is biologically inactive and considered inert. Nitrogen is slightly more soluble in fat than water, so people with more body fat will contain more nitrogen than a lean person weight for weight. During compression, when the pressure increases, the dissolved nitrogen in the tissues will also increase in pressure while the nitrogen volume is reduced. When the pressure is released during decompression, the dissolved nitrogen expands in the tissues until normal atmospheric pressure is restored. If the compression or decompression is small or slow, this has no biological consequences. The bends occur when the decompression is too rapid, as the expanding nitrogen, no longer dissolved, forms microbubbles, like the bubbles in champagne when the pressure is released as the cork is popped. When the nitrogen bubbles lodge in the joints, pain results. In rare cases the bends cause hyperventilation, and even death.

This bubble formation was observed by Robert Boyle in 1670 in snake blood when he exposed the reptile to a vacuum. At the time its significance was not realized.

Breathing Underwater

Diving has profound effects on our breathing, not due to an increase in pressure but to a different medium: viscous liquid water instead of gaseous air. Although we share an evolutionary link with fish, we are no longer capable of breathing via liquid mediums. Unlike fish, we are incapable of extracting oxygen efficiently from water, let alone our lungs being strong enough to ventilate with water for any appreciable time. When we dive below the water, we have to ensure that we have a constant supply of gaseous oxygen. This can be achieved by holding the breath or by pumping it in via umbilical tubing or from pressurized gas tanks carried on the back (scuba diving). Breathing through a snorkel allows for partial submersion underwater. The snorkel works by elongating our upper airways by several centimetres. The snorkel is positioned so that when we swim horizontally below the surface the snorkel tube will be raised above the water, allowing the diver to breathe. While the snorkel sounds like the ideal solution to underwater breathing, it suffers from a physiological limitation: as its length increases, its volume increases. This results in an increase in the so-called deadspace (after the German *Totraum*). With normal breathing, each breath contains waste gas left over from the previous breath. The inspired volume has to be large enough to account for the deadspace while providing enough fresh air to supply the tissues with adequate oxygen. Typically, 500 millilitres of exhaled breath may contain 120 millilitres of deadspace gas. This deadspace gas will have low oxygen and high CO_2 levels. Therefore, if the snorkel tube (extra deadspace), is too long the inspired volume will consist entirely of waste gas, and too little oxygen will reach the tissues. Swimming elephants can use their long trunks as natural snorkels, but they are adapted to having a snorkel for a nose.[22]

Holding the breath is the simplest way to swim underwater. This again has obvious limitations in that most of us can only hold our breaths for 1 to 2 minutes. With practice this can be extended to 3–4 minutes. However, in some people this can be 8–10 minutes. We all possess a dormant talent called the dive reflex, which means that if we submerge our faces in water while holding our breaths, we can hold it for much longer, as long as 50 per cent

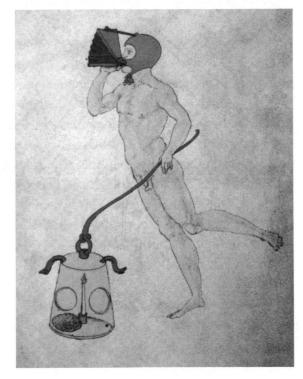

Diving apparatus designed by an anonymous Sienese engineer, *c.* 15th century. This drawing depicts a diver with bellows for breathing underwater and a watertight lamp with candle. The bellows would only allow a few minutes' submergence at most.

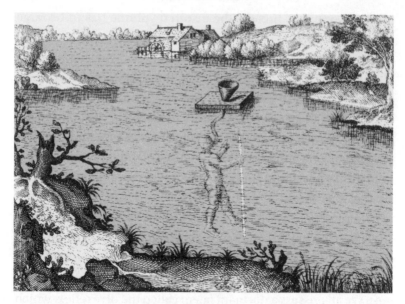

Fludd's Underwater Breathing Apparatus. The diver breathes through a
mask connected to a floating funnel allowing the diver to be mobile and stay
submerged just below the surface for extended times. From Robert Fludd,
*The metaphysical, physical technical history of the two worlds, namely the
greater and the lesser* (1617–21).

longer. This reflex is developed further in other diving mammals
such as seals, dolphins and whales. Breath holding has been practised for millennia by divers who collect sponges from the sea
bottom, particularly in the shallow Mediterranean Sea.

Descending below the water surface increases the external
pressure on the ribcage. As depth increases, so does the weight of
water above the diver (weighing around 1,024 kg per cubic metre);
the atmospheric pressure also increases. For every 10 metres (33 ft)
submerged the pressure increases by two atmospheres. Unlike in
air, this continues in a linear fashion, so at 20 metres it increases
to three atmospheres and at 30 metres (99 ft) to four atmospheres.
Physics dictates that as gas pressure increases, gas volume must
decrease. As a consequence, the gas volume in the lungs will
increase with depth, and the air also becomes denser, which
means it flows less well. Divers have to breathe harder to overcome the greater resistance resulting from greater density. The
gas has to be breathed at raised pressure, so divers often breathe

compressed air, or gas. At higher pressures gas can have biological effects not observed in uncompressed states. For example, when breathing nitrogen under pressure, below 20 metres (66 ft), it has effects on the nervous system and brain, resulting in nitrogen narcosis. At these pressures, nitrogen acts as an anaesthetic, leading to a drunken, confused state in the diver. It is sometimes called the Martini effect, as it feels like drinking alcohol on an empty stomach. To others it causes euphoria, so the narcosis is also called raptures of the deep. Thus for greater depths the nitrogen is replaced by helium (a heliox mixture), which like neon does not induce anaesthesia.

Austrian freediver Herbert Nitsch holds the record for free diving down to 253 metres (830 ft) in 2012. Freedivers hold their breath throughout the dive. Nitsch nearly died during this record attempt, as on his way back up 10 minutes into the dive, at a depth of 80 metres, he fell asleep due to nitrogen narcosis, and then as he reached a depth of 26 metres, his rescue team, seeing him unresponsive, lifted him rapidly to the surface, where he quickly revived. He went straight back underwater to try and decompress

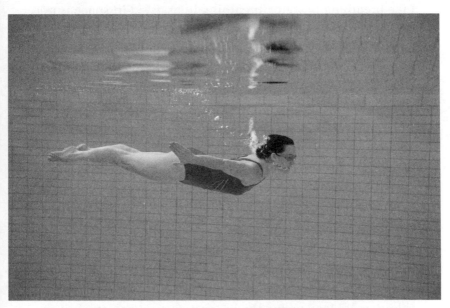

Swimming underwater while holding your breath can be an exhilarating experience.

properly, but it did not work, and he suffered from decompression sickness (the bends) and ended up in hospital in a coma for a few months. He eventually recovered fully. At this depth, the air in your lungs is so compressed that breathing becomes hard. It is only on the return to the surface that the air in the lungs expands back to normal.

Holding the breath has itself turned into an extreme discipline called static apnoea, in which a person submerged in water remains motionless while holding their breath. In 2014 Branko Petrović held his breath for 11 minutes and 54 seconds, and in 2013 Natalia Molchanova for 9 minutes and 2 seconds, both world records for breath-holding using air. If the nitrogen is substituted with oxygen, the breath-holding time increases dramatically. By breathing pure oxygen for around 20 minutes before his attempt, Budimir Šobat, in 2018, was able to hold his breath for 24 minutes and 11 seconds.

Breathing Above and Beyond

Like breathing in water, breathing unassisted in space is not possible. Space itself contains very little gas, let alone oxygen, and neither does the atmosphere of the moon or our neighbouring planets. On Earth the atmosphere ends and space begins at the Kármán line. Humans entering space must take along with them their own oxygen supplies, whether inside a spacesuit or in the International Space Station (ISS). Above the Earth's surface the weaker gravity has an effect on breathing.[23] Microgravity can make breathing a little difficult, as the blood flow and distribution of each breath within the lungs is different to that seen in full gravity. Gravity alters the structure of the lungs in an effect known as the 'slinky effect', and the way the blood flows around them. On Earth, we are one of the few animals that stands upright, so gravity influences the top of the lungs differently to their base. The top is ventilated differently to the bottom of the lungs, as is the distribution of blood within the lungs. This results in efficient gas exchange, as blood flows only to the areas of the lung that are being ventilated with fresh air. In space these differences disappear. Unlike at altitude, the lungs do not adapt to space, and on return lung function is unaffected. This is all good news for later missions to Mars and beyond: breathing should not be affected by space travel.

In space, humans must breathe in synthetic atmospheres in pressurized cabins. Before going to the Moon, the first Apollo astronauts had to test their space capsules and life support systems. The problem is to provide sufficient oxygen to support life while removing the excess carbon dioxide created by the astronauts. Oxygen is highly flammable and can be supplied from pressurized cylinders or from cryogenic liquid oxygen. In *Apollo 1*, the engineers decided to fill the launch capsule with 100 per cent oxygen, as this would maximize the amount of oxygen available for the planned long flights to the moon. On the launch pad an electrical spark ignited the cabin oxygen and the three crew members were fatally incinerated.

On the ISS, which has been continuously occupied for more than twenty years, a more sophisticated approach was required, as supplying the ISS with bottled oxygen would have been too expensive. So, a system to recycle the oxygen was developed. Oxygen can be easily generated from water, which is split into its component parts, hydrogen and oxygen, by passing through it an electric current, electrolysis. The ISS is exposed to direct sunlight for a good proportion of its orbit, so its solar panels can provide the necessary electricity. The oxygen so generated is added to the cabin atmosphere, breathed by the astronauts and converted and exhaled as carbon dioxide. The oxygen can be recycled again, this time making use of the hydrogen generated from the electrolysis of water. When hydrogen and carbon dioxide react, methane (CH_4) and water are formed. This water is then recycled for electrolysis. Recycling water from showers can be used to generate around 5–9 kilograms of oxygen needed per day for ISS. The body also excretes water in exhaled breath, as water vapour, in sweat, and in urine and faeces. All of this water can be recovered and recycled.

The breathing of space station astronauts is little affected by their stay in space, but they do suffer from one small but common problem: waking up gasping. In microgravity exhaled air does not automatically rise and mix with room air as it does on Earth, so in the ISS the exhaled gas remaining around the person increases the carbon dioxide levels. If allowed to build up, this will wake the sleeping person abruptly. Care is now taken to ventilate resting areas.

On Mars there are two major options to supply oxygen: one is to extract frozen water from the soil at the north and south poles, for instance, and use electrolysis and recycling, as on the ISS. The other solution is to split the plentiful CO_2 in the atmosphere into carbon and oxygen. Mars's atmosphere, although less dense than Earth's, is 96 per cent CO_2. The cultural impact of leaving Earth and colonizing another planet is immense and the consequences unimaginable, but this future depends on our ability to be able to breathe comfortably over a sustainable period. Breathing, then, is central to the destiny of humankind.

Although high oxygen levels are toxic, in some cases, if breathed under high-pressure conditions (hyperbaria), for instance while the person sits in a chamber, they may be beneficial. The first hyperbaric chambers were built even before the discovery of oxygen when in 1662 a British physician, one Dr Henshaw, built a pressurized airtight chamber he called a 'domicilium'.[24] Modern hyperbaric chambers are made of reinforced steel. One indication for breathing pure oxygen in a pressurized chamber is to treat carbon monoxide poisoning. The rationale for the therapy is that the oxygen will displace the tightly bound CO quicker when under excess pressure. Often though, by the time the affected person has been transported to the chamber, the poisoning has already cleared. High oxygen may have negative neurological effects, so it is not recommended lightly for CO poisoning.[25] Hyperbaric oxygen therapy (HBT) has been used to treat burns and aid wound healing and soft tissue sports injuries. The evidence for its effectiveness is sparse, so HBT seems to be more a whimsy than a necessity. The same can be said for the treatment of multiple sclerosis and cancer with HBT. Indeed, high oxygen pressures can cause convulsions, known as the Paul Bert effect, as seen in divers. If experienced underwater, these can be fatal. Oxygen toxicity on the nervous system has been known for a long time, as described by the French zoologist and physiologist Paul Bert, who exposed a wide range of flora and fauna to high oxygen levels, publishing his findings in *La Pression barometrique* in 1878. He concluded: 'an increase in oxygen tension above its normal value in ordinary air seemed to bring no advantage . . . When any difference is noticeable it is in the favour of normal air.'[26]

BREATHING AT ALTITUDES above and below sea level requires acclimatization. At raised altitudes, such as mountains, where oxygen mass is lower, breathing becomes more difficult and limits life to an upper level of 5,000 metres (16,400 ft). Contrary to this, in low-lying regions where the oxygen mass is enriched, there is little change to normal breathing, and it helps only those with impaired breathing and those who suffer from chronic lung disease. Artificially increasing the atmospheric pressure leads to its own problems with the respiratory system. The history of the bends has developed as our technology has improved over the past few centuries, first in digging supports for bridges and then with diving technology. This allowed us to dive ever deeper, whether for sport, as in free-diving, or for professional reasons such as servicing the oil and gas installations on the seabed. Finally, whether it is high in the Earth's orbit, on the Moon or the planet Mars, we will need in the future to build and maintain synthetic atmospheres, developing and refining the technology to recycle exhaled carbon dioxide and excreted water back into oxygen. Eventually breathing in space will be no different to breathing on Earth at sea level.

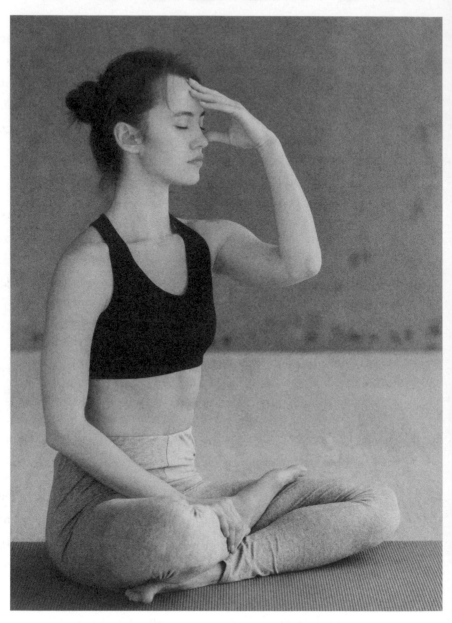

Woman practising yoga, in the Anuloma Viloma pose.

SEVEN

BREATHING FAST AND SLOW: BREATHE IN, BREATHE OUT

B reathing techniques are in common use nowadays. These are linked closely with meditation, evolving through religious beliefs and doctrine. Many are considered beneficial, providing a feeling of well-being, enhancing relaxation and thereby reducing stress. The link between meditation and breathing is steeped in Eastern tradition, originating in China and India over the last millennium. In Western culture many breathing techniques have been adopted only recently and free of religious beliefs, based on psychological theory and included in therapeutic regimes for treating conditions such as anxiety. The basis of the Eastern breathing techniques is to control the rate of breathing and quieten the breather's state of mind, while the newer Western techniques are based on paced breathing.[1]

Paced Breathing

Paced breathing is used in the treatment of psychological conditions where overbreathing or erratic breathing causes distress and ill feeling.

A common condition linked with psychological well-being is primary dysfunctional breathing (PDB), which is characterized by erratic breathing and is almost exclusively linked to a person's raised emotional state, which can be triggered by a variety of reasons, such as anxiety, suppressed anger or grief.[2] The main symptoms are breathlessness, dizziness and heart palpitations.

197

Often the person will hold their breath for short periods or breathe rapidly through their mouth instead of their nose. There is usually no abnormal lung pathology and the abnormal breathing is driven by the person's emotional status. The link between emotional status and the control of breathing is exaggerated. The raised emotional state overrides the normal respiratory rhythm, which tends to unbalance the blood oxygen, carbon dioxide and acid levels. While hyperventilating (overbreathing), the person will often focus on their breathing, leading to an increased rate, making things worse. It seems that the person loses the ability to see that they are overreacting to the situation.[3] In fact, it is believed that in PDB attentional control and emotional regulation are compromised. To slow the breathing, it is normal to divert the person's attention away from their breathing and calm them down, with the notion of disengaging the emotion from the breathing. With PDB this does not always work, but eventually the panic will subside and breathing returns to normal.

Hyperventilation syndrome (HVS) was first medically described in the 1930s but became apparent during the Second World War in Royal Air Force pilots, especially those not receiving supplemental oxygen. At higher altitudes, hypoxia would stimulate hyperventilation, resulting in light-headedness, feelings of unreality, anxiety, paraesthesia (a sensation of tingling), visual disturbances (such as blurring and loss of vision) and palpitations: a disturbing set of feelings and sensations when piloting a plane.[4] Today aircrew can suffer from hyperventilation while flying. This is due to physical disturbances such as air turbulence, motion sickness or whole-body vibration, but the most common cause is anxiety or emotional stress. This reaction is also seen in commercial airline passengers as well, often during take-off and landing, and when flying through turbulence. Outside of aviation the occurrence of HVS is also associated with abrupt emotional reactions, usually in adolescents in response to stressful situations. Overbreathing causes the carbon dioxide levels in the blood to fall to low levels. This is generally good for the tissues but not for the brain, which is bathed in cerebrospinal fluid (CSF). The carbon dioxide levels in the CSF alter the acid balance around the brain. When CO_2 levels are low the CSF become less acidic, which produces a feeling of giddiness and unwellness, which trigger the subject to overbreathe further. A simple cure for overbreathing is to ask the person to rebreathe into a bag (paper or plastic). This rebreathing tends to raise the CO_2 levels, effectively restoring the acid balance in the CSF, with the breathing returning to normal and the emotional episode usually subsiding after a minute or so. One has to be cautious when treating people exhibiting hyperventilation with 'paper-bag breathing', because if there is an underlying pathological reason for hyperventilation, such as during an asthma attack, prolonged breathing into a paper bag can be fatal: the breathing may cease altogether through asphyxiation, lack of oxygen.

The Buteyko breathing method was developed by the Ukrainian physician Konstantin Buteyko (1923–2003), who studied yoga and reasoned that hyperventilation in respiratory disease lowers the carbon dioxide levels in the blood. He further reasoned that lower CO_2 levels caused many of the symptoms associated with chronic respiratory disease, such as asthma, COPD and some sleep disorders. He advocated that it was possible to train people to breathe more slowly and raise their blood carbon dioxide levels to normal. One method of training includes taping the mouth shut while sleeping. Learning the Buteyko technique takes time and dedication, requiring two sessions per day. In asthmatics the technique has been shown to slightly reduce the symptoms and bronchodilator use. It does not alter the asthma itself but does provide a psychological way to control breathing.[5]

The Feldenkrais Method was developed by the Israeli Moshe Feldenkrais (1904–1984), who authored a book in 1942 about his ideas of linking well-being, posture and breathing. He states, 'Good breathing . . . means good posture, just as good posture means good breathing,' an aphorism reminiscent of breathing practice in yoga. Breathing and posture are linked through the mechanical connectivity of the chest and spine. Behind this method is the notion that through using different breathing cycles, such as 'inhale, pause, exhale, pause', irregular breathing disappears and the body learns to effectively enhance the person's health or well-being.[6]

Pilates is another popular fitness method which advocates changes in breathing, designed by the German Joseph Hubertus Pilates (1883–1967), who called his technique 'Contrology'. He developed a series of exercises while he was a prisoner of war during the First World War. The ethos of his system was that the body is actively regulated and controlled by the mind, and exercise redressed the effects of chronic physical inactivity. Breathing is one of the six central tenets of Pilates, along with concentration, control, centre, precision and flow.[7] The practitioner is encouraged to inhale and exhale deeply while maintaining a rigid posture to increase oxygen uptake and improve circulation. Joseph Pilates advised people to 'squeeze out the lungs as they would wring a wet towel dry'. Today Pilates is practised by millions of people worldwide.

Tai chi, and Qigong, have been practised for over 5,000 years, evolving under the Chinese Taoist system following the doctrine of improving general mental and physical health through gentle exercise. This form of meditation includes control of posture,

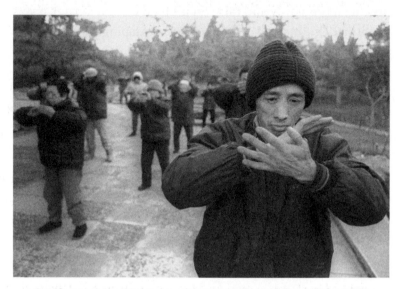

People practising Qigong breathing exercises in Beijing's Ritan Park.

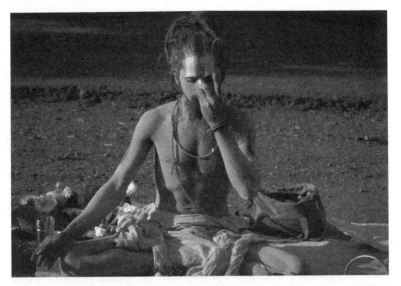

Sadhu, or wandering Hindu monk, meditating and Pranayama breathing in Madhya Pradesh, India.

movement, sound and breathing techniques. The techniques aim to cultivate and enhance qi (chi), the vital energy of life in Chinese traditional medicine, and are practised widely worldwide. Slow nasal breathing is encouraged. While thinking about breathing, the practitioner is encouraged to exhale into the urge to breathe as it occurs. Placing the tongue on the roof of mouth reinforces this method of breathing. This controlled breathing aids in relaxation and meditation. Some practitioners raise their arms while inhaling and lower them during exhalation. These breathing exercises seem to improve oxygen and carbon dioxide exchange while promoting calmness, which promotes well-being and reduced breathlessness in people with chronic lung diseases such as asthma and COPD.[8]

According to traditional Chinese medicine, hiccups occur when the stomach qi or the body's vital energy is disturbed or weakened. When the disturbed qi 'offends' the diaphragm, the lungs hiccup as a result.[9] Therefore, the traditional Chinese cure for hiccups is herbs and heat-clearing mixtures (containing ground scorpion and earthworm powders). These work by causing the rebellious qi to descend from the diaphragm and for the lung qi to disperse, while at the same time promoting the secretion of the body's fluids.

One widely popular form of meditation linked to posture and breathing is yoga. Yoga in its modern form has long roots that are associated with the history of alchemy and occultism of medieval India (tenth to eleventh century), and is now part of Hindu culture.[10] It is also linked to tantric ideas concerning the immobilization of semen in males. Today yoga has been systemized into a form of physical well-being and split between the practice of asana, postural exercise, and pranayama, breathing exercises, which are both based on the idea of creating a holistic well-being. Yoga was popularized in the West in the early twentieth century by practitioners from India and scholars of Oriental studies. Sir John Woodroffe (1865–1936), a specialist in Indian law and a don at the University of Oxford, published studies on Indian philosophy under his pseudonym Arthur Avalon and published two books: *The Serpent Power* and the *Garland of Letters*. *The Serpent Power* was based on a translation of a 1550 Sanskrit text accompanied by a detailed commentary of its philosophy. The Serpent power describing the energy released during the practice.

Yoga was popularized by the early practitioner Swami Vivekananda, who travelled around the United States in 1893. He gave talks on yoga, explaining its spiritual basis and alluding to its practice through references to anatomy and physiology. Through these lectures Yoga gained credibility and the process of 'medicalization' began. These views were further strengthened as they coincided with the health reform movement gaining popularity in the USA at the end of the nineteenth century.

Today there are many forms of yoga, but they are based on four types of practice, Karma yoga, work done selflessly, Jnana yoga, book knowledge as well as the truths of life, Bhakti yoga, devotion to a non-specific supreme force, and Raja yoga, spiritual growth. Yoga is thought to engender well-being by restoring an imbalance between instinct and intellect, an imbalance in the body's energy (*Prana*), as stated by one yoga advocate, 'the manifestations of a distracted state are mental anguish, tremors, rough and erratic breathing, and general nervousness' Patanjali Yoga Sutras (Chapter 1, Verse 31).

Among these various aspects of yoga practice, there are several breathing exercises called *pranayama* (*prana* = 'vital force', or 'life energy' also conveying breath, and *ayama* = 'to prolong', in Sanskrit). In most cases yogic breathing should be slow and deep with exhalation paused and lasting twice as long as inhalation (providing a 1:2 ratio). When practising Kapalabhati, the exhalation is more forced, and breathing rates climb to 60–120 breaths per minute, which is more akin to panting seen in animals. The practice of these breathing exercises are best pursued in the early morning or two hours after a meal, in a cool, quiet, well-ventilated room. They are usually done with the eyes closed, while sitting or standing erect. To conduct these exercises correctly requires the person to relax and focus on their breathing. It is this focus that leads to a clear mind and a sense of well-being.

These breathing exercises require inward concentration and thought, as breathing is directed through specific nostrils. The idea is that each nostril possesses a different function, just the left and right hemispheres of the brain are thought to host different temperaments. Breathing through the right nostril generates heat and is representative of being active both mentally and physically. This is called *surya anuloma viloma* (where *surya* means sun and *anuloma viloma* is inhale-exhale in Sanskrit). Left nostril breathing (termed *chandra anuloma viloma*) is associated with the moon (*chandra* = moon in Sanskrit). This nostril has a cooling effect, and consequently promotes more considered and thoughtful activities. The idea that the moon and sun provide a natural balance bound in a cyclical relationship, just as night and day are opposites and appear after one another, permeates many cultures.[11]

Breathing through alternate nostrils is practised by using the fingers and thumbs, using them to block one nostril at a time. This way single-nostril breathing can be practised for 20–30 minutes. Alternate nostril breathing, known simply as *anuloma-viloma*, can be performed this way also. Alternate nostril breathing for short periods is restful and promotes relaxation and meditation, but if practised too long it can raise the blood pressure and have a negative influence on health.

Creating sound while exhaling is a further yoga technique called *bhramari pranayama*, or bumblebee breathing. As the name suggests, to practise this particular breathing requires the creation of a low humming sound in the throat during exhalation. While exhaling, the ears are blocked, which allows the breather to feel the low frequency rumble generated in the oropharynx (throat). It is the inward concentration of this vibration that helps to focus and relax the mind. Another variation on this is *udgeeth pranayama*, where, after a deep inhalation, the chant 'Om' is made during each exhalation.

The American scientist Jon Kabat-Zinn (1944–) was an early advocate of using meditation and mindfulness to promote wellness. In his 1991 book *Full Catastrophe Living: Using Wisdom of Your Body and Mind to Face Stress, Pain and Illness* he describes the basic premise of relaxation through posture and stress relief by slow breathing, known as mindfulness-based stress reduction (MBSR). He defines meditation thus: 'Meditation is really a nondoing. It is the only human endeavour . . . that does not involve trying to get somewhere else but . . . being where you already are.'[12] Describing the breathing exercises, he states, 'we feel it come in and we feel it go out'; in other words, practitioners concentrate on slow breathing for ten minutes, once a day, distracting their thoughts away from the everyday, and helping to refocus their thoughts inward. The rationale behind the breathing exercises and daily practice is to reduce stress by concentrating on slow breathing, leaving behind your worries.

Slow breathing is part of many Western and Eastern meditation traditions. A common slow breathing rate is around 10 per minute, or one every six seconds. Slower rates are achievable but are at best uncomfortable and at worst detrimental to maintaining adequate tissue oxygenation. The main physical effect of slow breathing is to reduce arterial blood pressure. Thus, apart from for meditation, slow breathing has been used to treat people with high blood pressure or hypertension.[13]

The control of blood pressure is just as important as a constant supply of oxygen to the organs. The body is delicately balanced to meet both of these demands. Located in our necks and closely associated with our carotid arteries (which supply the head and brain with blood) are sensing bodies that detect blood pressure and oxygen levels. These sensors provide feedback to the brain, which then acts accordingly by increasing or decreasing breathing rate, heart rate or vasoactivity (contractility of the blood vessels). This response is known as the baroreflex. Slow breathing works by altering the baroreflex sensitivity and reducing the activity of

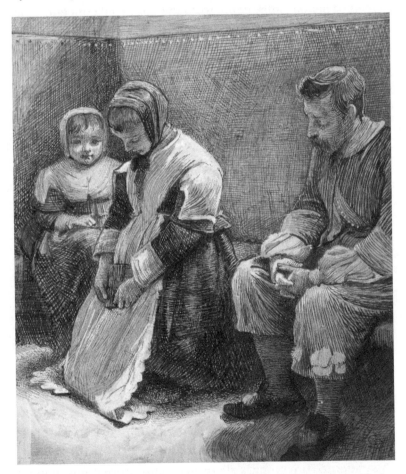

George J. Pinwell, *Prayer Is the Christian's Vital Breath*, 1866, printers block, drawing. Communal prayer alters breathing, usually by slowing the breathing rate.

the controlling nervous system.[14] Thus meditative practices that engender slow breathing will alter blood pressure, as will yoga mantras and rosary prayers. Their practice slows breathing and will lower blood pressure and anxiety. The act of prayer by rosary could be considered a health practice as well as a religious practice, having both physiological and psychological effects.[15] The practice of other yogic breathing techniques such as Ujjayi, where the duration of inspiration and expiration are controlled separately in addition to a slow breathing rate, increase the work of breathing but do not seem to alter the cardiovascular system. The perceived benefits may come from the increased concentration required in its performance.[16] Other forms of vocalization, such as speaking, may not alter blood pressure, but can change the heart rate: breathing and heart rate have been shown to synchronize during poetry recitals, for example, with the rhythm of the reciter's breathing reflecting the structure of the poem.[17]

For many cultures breathing is a spiritual phenomenon, associated with life and death. Indigenous Australians name their breath-related spirit *wau-wau*, which leaves the body upon death to become a spirt of nature. Similarly, when asleep or unconsciousness, the spirit is thought to leave the body, but only temporarily, with its return marked by wakening.

Patterned Breathing

During childbirth, controlled or patterned breathing techniques are advocated to help mothers manage pain and shorten the duration of labour.[18] The principle behind this idea is that the very act of thinking about breathing, by breathing in deeply and matching exhalation with exertion, helps to distract the mother and so reduces her perception of pain severity. Breathing this way can only be performed for short periods, as it is hard work, so starting the breathing exercises too early in the birth can increase fatigue.[19] This patterned breathing is also called Lamaze breathing, named after the French obstetrician Fernand Lamaze (1891–1957), who after travelling to Russia and the Ukraine in 1951 witnessed the use of patterned breathing to control pain. Dr Lamaze developed his patterned breathing techniques in his Paris clinic, where the American Marjorie Karmel, who found herself pregnant in Paris and had read Grantley Dick-Read's book *Childbirth without Fear*, sought out Lamaze. On returning to the USA in 1959, she published a book about her experience, *Thank You, Dr Lamaze*. At this time Elisabeth Bing (1914–2015), a German physiotherapist who had left Germany to avoid Nazi persecution and emigrated to the USA in 1933, developed an interest in obstetrics and became a proponent of natural childbirth. Bing was keen to learn more about Lamaze's methods, but could not obtain funds to travel to Paris. In 1959, when Bing saw the book, she contacted Karmel's publisher, hoping to get in touch with her. Two weeks after the book was published, Karmel contacted Bing, asking her if she would take on the role of educating women in the technique. Through wide publicity on the radio and television, the idea of patterned breathing was popularized.

Strangely, the idea of using patterned breathing was first published in the USA 54 years earlier by the American dentist William Gibson Arlington Bonwill. He was convinced that he could perform minor surgery without the need for nitrous oxide, instead pain relief was achieved through rapid breathing. He published his views in 1880 in a paper titled 'Rapid Breathing as a Pain Obtunder in Minor Surgery, Obstetrics, the General Practice of Medicine and Dentistry'. Unlike Dr Lamaze, when Dr Bonwill visited Russia in 1897, he went there to promote his rapid breathing technique rather than to learn it.[20]

An especially useful but unusual form of breathing was developed in Rancho Los Amigos, California. In the 1940s this was a hospital housing poliomyelitis patients with 'pronounced poliomyelitic impairment of the respiratory muscles', who required artificial ventilation.[21] These patients made a remarkable discovery: they found that they could breathe ventilator-free for a few hours if they gulped air. This so-called frog breathing involves first taking a normal inspiration to fill the lungs, and then gulping and swallowing more air via the mouth. The air is trapped in the lungs by the glottis. By taking ten to twenty gulps, the amount of air in lungs can be increased to normal or even a raised volume. The name of the patient who discovered this form of breathing is not known, but soon many of their fellow patients learnt how to do it, and their time off the ventilator rose from just 2–25 minutes a day to 2–3 hours. The change to their quality of life was huge; the patients' morale soared. They were able to sit up in bed rather than lying flat, and could cough and expectorate freely. Having more air to expire also meant they could talk louder and for longer. Frog breathing, or glossopharyngeal breathing or insufflation, to give it its correct name, is now widely advocated in many cases where the respiratory muscles are weak, such as Duchenne muscular dystrophy or after paralysis from injury to the cervical spinal cord.[22] This extreme form of breathing has been adopted by free-divers, who call it 'stacking'. Before diving, they first fill their lungs to maximum (called the total lung capacity), and then rapidly frog-breathe, adding a few litres of extra air into their lungs. These can make the diver feel faint and holding the extra air can be uncomfortable, but it seems nothing in free diving is free.

Emotion and Breathing

While Charles Darwin is famous for his first book *On the Origin of Species*, which expostulates his idea of evolution by means of natural selection, it was followed in 1871 by his next book, *The Descent of Man, and Selection in Relation to Sex*. This work attempted to apply evolution to the human condition and society. It was one of the first books to systematically review human behaviour and psychology in terms of evolution. Darwin was aware of the dangers of upsetting Victorian society, given the subject of the book, so he asked his daughter Henrietta to edit and sanitize the text. During its writing he began to try and catalogue human emotions and see if they could be found in animals. These observations were originally supposed to occupy a few pages of this second book but grew to such an extent that they soon warranted a whole book of their own, so in 1872 they were published in *The Expression of the Emotions in Man and Animals.* In this book Darwin classified emotions such as anger and fear as separate entities, unlike today, where emotions are considered a spectrum of expressions with differing intensities. Darwin associated different breathing rates and patterns with different emotions, stating that 'Terror causes the body to tremble. The breathing is hurried. The heart beats quickly, wildly and violently.' In other emotions he observed interrupted breathing: suffering and weeping manifested as 'The mouth is widely opened with the lips retracted in a peculiar manner, which causes it to assume a squarish form; the gums or teeth being more or less exposed. The breath is inhaled almost spasmodically.' While weeping the breathing becomes stuttered, and the nose becomes filled with mucus and lacrimal fluid or tears. Lacrimal fluid drains from the eyes via the lacrimal canals (Latin: *lacrimal canaliculi*), which pass into the left and right nasolacrimal canals, which themselves pass into the nasal cavity just above the roof of the mouth. Normally this fluid produced continuously by the lacrimal glands, located under the upper eyelids, goes unnoticed, but whenever we cry excess fluid floods our eyes and the front of our nose, which runs profusely. Often a crying person is offered a handkerchief to mop up the tears on their face and to blow their nose. This offer is not only seen as practical but as an act of kindness and a sign of empathy. After weeping, grief sets in, which Darwin characterizes as when 'The breathing becomes slow and feeble and is often interrupted by deep sighs.' With the fiercer emotions such as anger, the opposite is the case: 'The respiration is affected; the chest heaves, and the dilated nostrils quiver.'

Darwin draws on many of his own observations but also from two other observers: the French physician Louis Pierre Gratiolet, whose book *De la Physionomie et des mouvements d'expression*, was published posthumously in 1871, and the other the Scottish physician Sir Charles Bell, in his *Essays on the Anatomy and Philosophy of Expression as Connected with the Fine Arts* (1844). While Darwin extensively quoted these books, their views on the origin of species were completely opposed to his. Bell believed in religious creationism and countered the timeline of evolution with his own theory that while God had created animals at once, the conditions of the Earth were fluid instead and changed over time, instead of one single creation event, as described in Genesis.

The notion that emotion alters breathing is found throughout literature. Tennyson writes, 'sharp breaths of anger puffed her fairy nostrils out' in the poem 'Merlin and Vivien' in *Idylls of the King*. Giving us such expressions as 'breathing out vengeance' and 'fuming with anger', Shakespeare sums up the chief characteristics of rage as follows, in his play *Henry V*:

> In peace there's nothing so becomes a man,
> As modest stillness and humility;
> But when the blast of war blows in our ears,
> Then imitate the action of the tiger:
> Stiffen the sinews, summon up the blood,
> Then lend the eye a terrible aspect;
> Now set the teeth, and stretch the nostril wide,
> Hold hard the breath, and bend up every spirit
> To his full height! On, on, you noblest English. (III.1)

Often, we make single odd breaths, such as a sigh or a large single breath. Sighs are thought to serve a physiological function of clearing the lungs by every now and again expanding and stretching the airways. However, sometimes a sigh is a sign of disappointment. The American writer Minna Antrim (1861–1950) states, 'The drama of life begins with a wail and ends with a sigh.'

When we make noisy breaths, which occur when we exert ourselves, such as when we walk up a steep hill or climb steps, we describe them with words such as 'huff' and 'puff'. If someone is in a huff, they are usually in a bad mood and ill-tempered, which generally has nothing to do with their breathing. Words such as 'whiff', 'sniff' and 'snuff' are all breathing manoeuvres associated with the nose. A whiff is a smell gathered during a sniff. A sniff is a small tentative inhale, usually made to sample an odour. It requires the diaphragm to contract quickly in order to generate a sharp negative pressure and draw air turbulently through the nose. This allows the olfactory nerves to get a good sample of air. Sniffing also has an emotional relationship and is associated with a 'runny nose', a nose producing copious amounts of fluid, a mixture of tears and mucus. When someone has a cold and a blocked nose, sniffing is performed to unblock the nasal passages. Solvents and drugs can also be sniffed, such as glue and cocaine. Volatile glue and fine powders are carried quickly to the nasal tissues during a sharp sniff. The nasal membranes are thin and perfused profusely with blood, so are an ideal site for absorbing soluble substances.

Breathing patterns are automatic when responding to our metabolic needs but also subconsciously require modification as we are influenced by our emotional state, such as when we laugh, and our behaviour and social activities, like talking and playing musical instruments.[23] For the brain, talking provides a complex challenge, as this requires the coordination of the breathing muscles with those of the lips, tongue and face, in unison with the need to interrupt the timing, rhythm and pattern of breathing. Before we utter a word, we must subconsciously breathe in enough air to complete the sentence we have forming in our minds. As we talk, we integrate our breathing seamlessly with our speech. Speech is generated during bouts of prolonged exhalation interspersed by quick sharp inhalations. The words and associated sounds are generated first by the vibrating vocal cords in the larynx, passing via the throat to the mouth where they are shaped and modified by the tongue and lips to form individual syllables, which are then joined up to form words and sentences.

When someone is singing, the brain's control needs to be even more refined. With this extreme form of breathing the respiratory muscles of the throat, ribcage and diaphragm need to be closely coordinated and controlled. In this case both inspiration and expiration must be regulated according to the accompanying music received via the ears and auditory system. A further complication is that singing often involves an emotional slant, whether it be joy or sadness. If breathing becomes uncoordinated, the notes may not be reached or held, and the resulting song becomes jerky

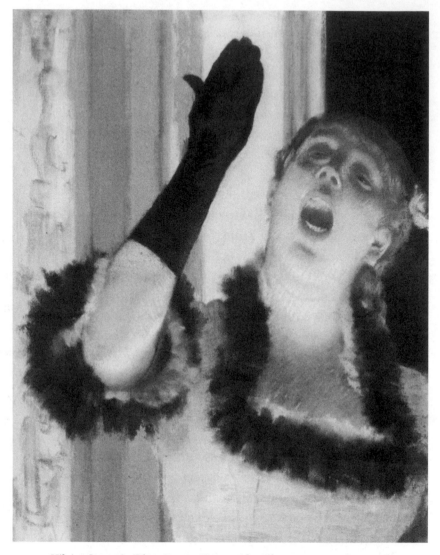

Hilaire Germain Edgar Degas, *Singer with a Glove*, 1878, pastel on canvas.
Mid-song, and with her hand aloft, the woman in Degas' painting expresses
the substantial effort and concentration required by singers.

and is unpleasant listening for the audience.[24] Singers learn to
'smuggle in the breath' and fill the lungs quickly when more air
is required, allowing elongation of expiration.[25]

As someone sings, their breathing must be controlled efficiently to prevent fatigue. The coordination of the rate at which
the expired flow is expelled and the passage of air across the vocal

cords generates the volume of the singing voice. This can only occur when the airflow is correct and the vocal cords are held in the right place.

Singing is considered entertainment but, as it exercises the respiratory system, it has many health benefits, improving the symptoms of chronic lung diseases such as COPD and asthma. Emotional benefits are also gained by singing, through the complex augmentation of the neural networks involved in the control of breathing and the coordination of the respiratory muscles. As a therapy, singing, whether solo, in a community setting or even as karaoke, provides physical improvements in health through exercising the breathing and aids good mental health in many ways.[26]

Our understanding of how we modulate the voice to sing was not understood until the early nineteenth century. In 1894 Ramsey Smith of the University of Edinburgh stated, 'The importance of correct breathing habits in singing is universally acknowledged, but the precise relation to breathing to singing has not been pointed out.'[27] In the context of breathing, singing interrupts its normal rhythm and lengthens the time between breaths. Singing is punctuated with quick inspirations and prolonged expirations, where the expired airflow is controlled with precision. This neural control is fed back through the auditory system of the singer. The singer then regulates their breathing to match the preconceived and correct musical notes and text. The notes and text have to be cued in advance. This is why most singers rehearse before singing in public. Studies have shown that singers do not require exceptional lung function and their rested quiet breathing is no different from that of non-singers. Frequent singing does allow the singer to learn to exhale more efficiently, so it is a change in ventilation that is important rather than a change in lung volume. As well as using the ribcage to breathe, singers make more use of abdominal breathing, and are able to desynchronize the two means of breathing, something untrained singers cannot do easily.[28] This extra control allows the generation of increased air pressure in the lungs, which in turn means a greater airflow through the larynx, thus increasing a person's vocal range.

Just listening to singing or music alters breathing. Studies have shown that music with a slow tempo, such as Ludwig Beethoven's Adagio from his Ninth Symphony (at 70 beats per minute), relaxes and slows breathing, much as meditation and chanting do. A fast tempo, such as Antonio Vivaldi's Presto from Estate, Concerto for violin orchestra and 'Summer' from the Four Seasons (150 beats per minute), can increase the breathing rate. In trained musicians this tempo effect is even more pronounced.[29]

Apart from singing and listening, playing music also alters breathing. The most obvious examples are wind instruments, which create sound through the vibrations caused by airflow through a restricted orifice. The flow is generated by the musician blowing or puffing air through the instrument under pressure.

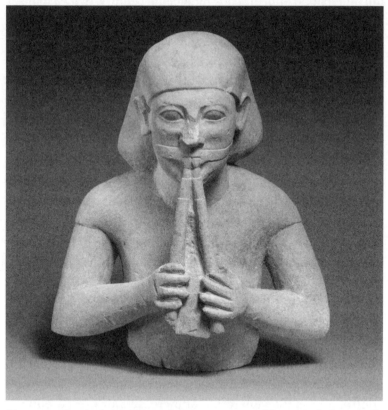

Limestone Cypriot bust of flute player, *c.* 575–500 BC (Cypro-Archaic period), using a *phorbia* (facial strap), which holds the flutes and prevents the cheeks inflating during play.

Playing wind instruments, like singing, has also been practised since antiquity, the earliest instruments being the first bone flutes from 40,000 years ago. Potential wind instruments are easy to find in nature: blowing through a hollow tube will create sound. A hollow branch or root will do, the didgeridoo being a good example. Many coastal areas are littered with conch shells, which when blown emit a deep resonant sound like that of a horn. Even a discarded cow horn will create a sound when blown through. The metallic wind instruments more familiar today appeared early in antiquity and were originally made of precious metals. (One fine ancient Egyptian example is the silver trumpet found in Tutankhamun's tomb from the fourteenth century BC.) Nowadays they are made of brass or wood. Surprisingly, the playing of musical instruments has not generated much scientific curiosity as to its effect on breathing or respiratory health.

With wind instruments, such as trumpets (classified as a brass instrument) or didgeridoos, or through a mouthpiece containing a reed, such as in an oboe (classified as a woodwind instrument), precise air control is required during expiration, as is the ability to generate sufficient mouth pressure to force air through the instrument tubing. Being able to generate the extra pressure to play wind instruments does not seem to require extraordinary lungs. Compared to other musicians, such as stringed instrument players, wind instrument players possess similar lung function, although there is some evidence that they may be more sensitive to lung infections in the upper airways, nasal catarrh and hoarseness.[30] Playing a wind instrument generally improves the sense of well-being, but if played for many years it may reduce lung volumes by a small amount, perhaps 200 to 300 millilitres, as a consequence of generating the extra pressure required.[31] While playing other instruments, the breathing rate can also be altered: for example, pianists will synchronize their breathing with their finger movements, the breathing unconsciously following the complex musical metres within the piece being performed.[32]

Before the sixteenth century the voice was considered separate to breathing and was known to emanate from the mouth but be

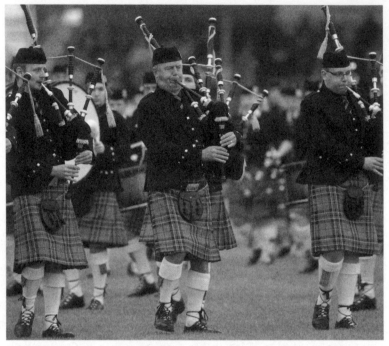

A group of pipers playing the bagpipes at the Highland Games, Scotland, 2017. Considerable respiratory effort is required to produce enough airflow to generate sound continuously.

created in the chest. The great Italian anatomist and surgeon Hieronymus Fabricius (1533–1619) was the first to link the larynx with the voice in his work *De larynge* (1615). Before this, the uncertainty about the location of the voice was reflected in the adjective 'ventriloquial', which means speaking through the abdomen. Since the mouth is not used, and the digestive system can generate sounds, it was assumed that a voice could be generated in this way. After Fabricius, in the early eighteenth century, two scientific views developed on how the voice was generated: one camp thought that the air acted on the vocal cords (or folds) just as a bow vibrates the strings on a violin. The other camp believed that the voice was generated in the same way a flute, horn or oboe create sound, via the reed vibrating as air flows across it. These musical analogies led to the word 'chord' being used originally to describe the laryngeal structures; this proved confusing, so instead 'cord' or 'fold' is used today.

The voice has three characteristics: loudness, pitch and timbre. Loudness or volume is regulated simply by changing the force of the expelled air, which increases the expired airflow rate. When you shout loudly, you can only do this for a few seconds at a time, whereas quieter sounds can be generated for many seconds longer. The voice's pitch changes with the length of the vocal cords, which generate sounds in the same way as violin strings. In males, who have longer vocal cords (2–2.5 cm, 0.8–1 in.), they vibrate like the violin's G string, while in women, who typically have shorter vocal cords (1.8 cm, 0.7 in.), they vibrate in a similar fashion to the E string. Males therefore have deeper voices than females. The length of vocal cords is changed by tension generated by the arytenoid cartilages: a low pitch is generated by relaxed cords and a high pitch by taut cords. This gives the possibility of generating a wide range of notes. Although the range men and

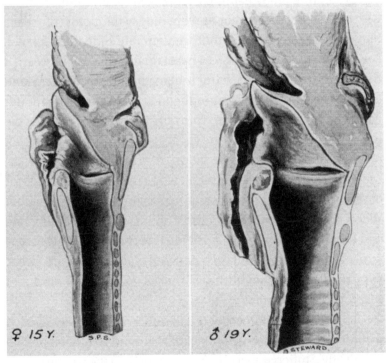

Growth changes of human larynx at puberty, 1965. The diameter of the glottis is 13 mm in the female and 22 mm in the male, deepening the male voice.

women can generate overlaps, men cannot generate the high notes women can reach. On the musical scale the voice ranges over three octaves, but with training this range can often be increased to four. In exceptional cases the range will be five octaves or more: examples of such singers are Mariah Carey, Prince and Yma Sumac.

Timbre or tone is dependent upon the movement of the expelled air through the cavities of the respiratory system, the moving air causing vibrations in these cavities depending on their size and structure. These have differences in tone similar to those between a violin and the larger cello. Trained singers can alter the harmonics of these vibrations and alter the qualities of their voice. When the vocal cords vibrate at 80–250 vibrations a second, a bass voice is heard. Vibrations from 100–350 per second give a baritone while 250–750 per second and higher produce a soprano.

By altering our breathing we can generate sounds, but it is with our mouth, lips, tongue and opening of the glottis (the space between the vocal cords) that we generate individual speech sounds. A word like 'sing' has a nasal quality that can be heard if the nose is held while the word is being pronounced. The sound 'ssss' in the word 'sip' is pronounced at the front of the mouth while the sound 'zzzz' in the word 'zip' is generated towards the rear, deep in the larynx and the vocal cords. The larynx can be felt to vibrate during the pronunciation of 'zzzz' but not 'ssss'.

Vocalization becomes difficult when metabolic demands for oxygen uptake and carbon dioxide expulsion become paramount. When we exercise vigorously, with an increased breathing rate and raised tidal volume, vocalization is very difficult and it is certainly strenuous to maintain a detailed conversation. Likewise, hypoxia due to higher altitudes makes vocalization hard and gasping can predominate.

Stuttering or stammering is a common but complex speech disorder thought to be experienced by around 70 million people worldwide. Stuttered speech is difficult for both the person speaking and listening. The speech can be repetitious, like 'ch, ch, chocolate', words can be prolonged or extended, like 'mmmanage', there can be blocks of pauses like 'a. a. apple', or there can be complete silence: many stutterers avoid talking, as this helps to steer clear of any social anxiety. While there are no cures for stuttering, there are ways of improving the stutter, which often include breathing exercises. One such technique is offered by the McGuire programme. This programme teaches the stutterer to talk by using the technique of 'pause, breathe, speak and release (expire)'. Once mastered, the pause becomes shorter and unnoticeable and many people regain their confidence enough to talk in public.

Speaking is a complex process requiring more than one hundred facial, respiratory and oropharyngeal muscles, all responding in the right order over a few milliseconds. The muscles are coordinated and timed by the nervous system, brain, cerebellum and basal ganglia. Stuttering is believed to be due to the neurotransmission of this timing becoming unsynchronized through faulty insulation of the myelin sheaths surrounding the nerves. Intact myelin sheaths are necessary for the perfect working of nerves. In addition to this, there is thought to be a problem in articulation and speech planning in Broca's area of the brain.

Our first detailed hints about how the brain independently generates its own rhythm comes from the humble goldfish. If the opportunity arises, take a close look at one breathing or gulping water. As in all fish, each gulp or mouthful of water is passed only one way, just backwards over the gills, where gas exchange takes place. Unlike air in the lungs, the movement of water isn't tidal, passing back and forth through the mouth. The water passes on through the gill flaps out into the surrounding water, a much simpler way to breathe. It was in 1931 that Edgar Douglas Adrian, Baron Adrian of Cambridge, noticed that regions of the isolated goldfish brain stem activity resonated at the same frequency as its breathing. The following year Adrian shared the Nobel Prize in Physiology or Medicine with Sir Charles Sherrington for their discoveries regarding the functions of neurons.

Today we still do not understand how breathing is regulated. One modern theory is the triple oscillator hypothesis. This hypothesis posits that each breathing phase is generated by three rhythmogenic circuits in the medulla. One neural circuit (oscillator) regularly and spontaneously creates bursts of activity, providing a regular breathing rate. A second circuit can inhibit this activity and slow the breathing rate, while a third can excite it. The balance among these three circuits generates and creates a rhythm. This rhythm then passes through other adjacent parts of the medulla, where it is translated into a breathing pattern; 'The activity of rhythm- and pattern-generating elements can be differentially tuned by various modulatory inputs to endow breathing with exquisite metabolic-, state- and behaviour-dependent control.'[33]

A major limitation of the throat is that it is not just a conduit for air but is also used for eating food and drinking liquids. When swallowed, food and drink enter the stomach via the oesophagus, which runs in parallel to the trachea (windpipe) and larynx. Air, food and liquid have all to pass through the larynx. To separate air from food and liquids, the epiglottis, a flap at the head of the larynx, can be closed. When we swallow the epiglottis shuts and the food and drink pass by into the oesophagus. When the swallow is over and the throat clears, the epiglottis opens and air is free to move back and forth between the atmosphere and the lungs. Sometimes, however, when we eat or drink and try to breathe or talk at the same time, the epiglottis may open at the wrong moment and fluid or food may enter the lungs. Fluid entering the lungs, or 'going the wrong way', makes you cough and splutter. Most people have experienced this sensation and it is an unpleasant one. Fluid is easily removed by coughing, but solid food is another matter, as hard food can become lodged in the airways with grave consequences.

The Scottish physician Peter Gilroy reported in 1831 a case study of a forty-year-old women, Mrs N., who in August 1826 was seized with a sudden and violent fit of coughing while eating her dinner. After recovering, she told her concerned friends that 'a chicken bone had gone wrong, and still was tickling in her chest.' All she could feel the next day was a slight tickling cough. The cough never receded, and she was bled twice as way of reducing the symptoms. By 13 September, around five weeks later, Mrs N. was bedbound and unable to move freely, as the pain in her upper sternum was severe if she raised her shoulder or coughed. The bone fragment had lodged in her trachea and the surrounding tissue had become infected. The wound festered and Mrs N. became feverish. Finally, on 29 October, she died, exhausted by 'pain, irritation and discharge'. Physicians could offer no treatment at this time. At the autopsy, they found the small piece of bone in the right lung. Weighing a paltry 0.4 grams, it was lodged in the trachea and protruded into a large smelly pus-filled abscess weighing around 570 grams.[34]

Other food that can impede breathing are nuts, particularly peanuts, which if they pass into the trachea can drop straight down the right carina and get lodged in a small airway, blocking a lobe or large section of the lung. This causes breathlessness in the short term. The peanut can decompose, which may cause infection. In children death has been caused by swallowing whole grapes. A grape is a flexible but rigid structure and if swallowed by a young child can lodge in the trachea and completely block the airways, causing asphyxiation. This leads to the guidance that all young children should be given halved or sliced grapes. There are documented cases of seeds falling into the lungs and germinating: in 2012 newspapers across the globe reported that while performing an endoscopy on a 28-year-old patient, a Russian doctor found a small fir-tree seedling growing in the man's airways.

Fragranced Breath

The air we breathe is never pure and contains many thousands of compounds, many of which we can detect using our sense of smell. If these smells are pleasant, we take enhanced breaths; if they are unpleasant, we do the opposite and refrain from breathing. The sense of smell or olfaction is a major function of the respiratory system. The smell-sensing tissues are located in the nose, where they are best exposed to airborne chemicals. One could argue that they are tasting the air; in fact, the senses of taste and smell are intimately linked. The sense of smell is seated in the upper respiratory tract and the chambers behind the two nares, or nostrils, are home to the sense of smell. Here special sensory nerves project from the base of the brain through the base of the skull into the roof of the nasal cavity. While these sensors work all the time, it is only when we become conscious of a smell that we interrupt our breathing. When we do, we stop and take a sniff, a special inspiration, whereby a sharp intake of air is drawn rapidly into the nose. Sometimes three or four small sniffs occur in quick succession before we exhale and return to normal breathing. The sniff is generated by creating negative pressure in the thorax, so that atmospheric air rushes quickly through the nose, creating turbulent airflow across the smell sensors. Most odours are not produced by a single compound but result from combinations of molecules: the smell of chocolate, for instance, is a combination of hundreds of odorant molecules, just like an expensive perfume or the fragrance from a rose.

We are capable of differentiating between hundreds of smells and endless combinations of odorants. Perfumes are a good example of this. The highest-quality perfumes are complex mixtures of odorant molecules mixed in very precise ratios, designed to be unique, subtle and enduring. This way we can tell the difference between Chanel No. 5 and J'adore by Dior. If we don't like a smell, we 'turn up our nose' and avoid it by holding our breath. Alternatively we hold our nose, pinching it between our fingers, holding the nares shut and breathing through our mouths. Luckily, our mouths do not possess a sense of smell, but can taste odours instead, which when foul can make us feel like gagging or vomiting. Not only can we smell the difference between coffee and tea, but we can distinguish the strength of a smell; it can have a whiff or hint of fragrance or be overpowering. Wine provides both a fragrance and a taste, and it is the combination of these that makes the drink pleasant.

We can temporarily lose our sense of smell when we have a cold, an upper respiratory tract infection (URTI), when the nose becomes blocked with thickened mucus that runs from the nose.

Head of an Arabian mare that shows its wide, flared nostrils, which expand or contract especially in exertion. Adapted from Lady Wentworth, *The Authentic Arabian Horse* (1945).

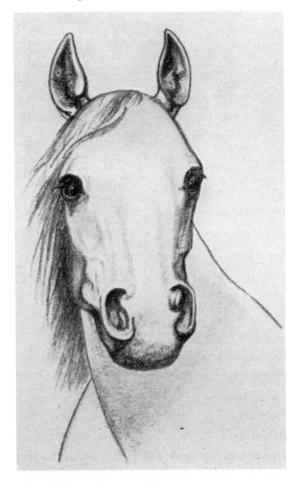

This prevents the odorant molecules reaching the smell sensors. In certain conditions the sense of smell can be lost completely, a condition called anosmia. This can result from physical trauma to the head or face in which the link between the nose and brain is broken. People with Parkinson's disease, dementia and some brain tumours can become anosmic. When we age, we lose our sense of smell, along with having an increased propensity towards breathlessness. Many smokers experience a reduced sense of smell and taste as the tobacco smoke destroys the sensory nerve endings.

We remember smells, as they can evoke a full range of emotions from fear through to happiness. Certain smells can even remind us of times and places long gone, for instance of our

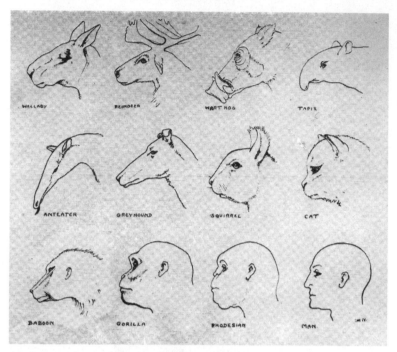

The snout is elongated in animals that need it to reach their food and short in species that can grasp food with their forelimbs. Composite illustration, from Sir Victor Negus, *The Biology of Respiration* (1965).

childhood. Thus breathing and the sense of smell play a key role in our lives. Without this sense, depression can result, and we can be put off the act of eating when the taste of food is either transformed for the worse or lost completely.

Drugs and Chemical Breathing

Volatile substances are molecules that can be carried in the air. Apart from stimulating the smell receptors, these molecules can cross from the lungs into the blood and have other effects on the body. They may provide anaesthesia or relief from pain and cold symptoms. Many of these compounds are produced by natural plants, while others are manufactured drugs. Plants placed in a room are said to freshen the air, and while they do not alter breathing, the small number of volatile molecules emitted by the plants provides a subtle lift to the occupants' mood and sense of well-being. Add in flowers and the visual stimulus improves the senses further.

There are some plants that influence breathing by emitting pungent vapours. One medicinal product with a mixture of these plant-based breathing aids is a proprietary medication called Vicks VapoRub. Most people have come across this cold medication at some point in their lives. Vicks VapoRub is dabbed or smeared on the skin of the upper chest when suffering from a blocked nose (nasal congestion) or a chesty cough. It is a memorable experience because of the 'medicinal' and strong vapour arising from the gel. When the gel is warmed by body heat after being smeared on the skin, the vapour is released into the air, which when it enters the nose gives the sensation of being able to breathe more easily. This can relax the person and aid sleep. The vapour does not seem to have any other effect.

The formula was invented in the 1890s by Lunsford Richardson, a pharmacist from Greensboro, North Carolina. Its future was secured during the Spanish flu pandemic when sales soared to unprecedented levels, from $0.9 million in 1917 to $2.9 million in 1918. Ironically, Richardson died of the same flu in 1919. Although it did not offer a cure, the widely held belief at the time was that it prevented the flu. It did offer some relief, however, once the airways and lung became congested.

The emitted vapour contains menthol, eucalyptus and camphor oils, all three derived from plants. Menthol is extracted from the mint family, which includes peppermint and spearmint. Menthol also has a cooling effect when ingested, as it temporarily disrupts the function of the oral temperature sensors, thus fooling the senses further. A mint-fragranced breath is considered pleasant. If one is concerned about bad breath, for instance after drinking strong coffee, then unpleasant smells can be masked either by sucking menthol sweets or chewing gum containing menthol or mint. The market for these sweets and gums is huge, amounting globally to several billion u.s. dollars annually.

The other plant oil in the Vicks preparation is eucalyptus oil. This is extracted from the leaves of the eucalyptus plant, a group of flowering trees and bushes in the myrtle family. Most of the seven hundred species originate from Australia, but owing to its hardy nature it is now found growing across the world as an ornamental garden tree. In some locations, such as California, it is an invasive species that has become naturalized. Eucalyptus or gum trees have evergreen leaves that are dull and covered in oily glands, making them flammable, and are thought to contribute to the large bush fires that seasonally sweep across California and Australia. It is eucalyptol (1,8-cineole) in the form of eucalyptus oil that is the active extract and works by making breathing easier through loosening mucus in the lung airways. If this oil is added to hot water, the steam can be inhaled deeply into the lungs. This inhalation method can easily lead to an overdose. In large doses eucalyptol affects the central nervous system and in the worst cases the person can become comatose. In lower doses it can cause bronchospasm, nausea and vomiting. Often those breathing vaporized steam collapse face-down into the bowl of hot water and scald their faces.

Another fragrant member of the mint family is oregano (*Origanum vulgare*), which has been used to treat breathing problems since ancient times. Oregano, a European plant, was known by the ancient Greeks, who believed that it was created by Aphrodite, the goddess of love. The plant's name is derived from Greek (*oros*: mountain, and *ganos*: joy, so 'joy of the mountains'). It was popular and was added to food for its flavour and used as a medicine to prevent coughing and sore throats. Although it is still used today as a folk remedy against colds and upset stomachs in Greece, there is little evidence to support these health benefits, but it is still a great addition to any pizza.[35]

Rosemary (*Rosmarinus officinalis*, Latin derivation: *sea dew*), also related to mint, originates from Asia but is now a common garden plant and herb. It has a distinct pungent smell that is an admixture of pine and lemon. The ancients conferred the plant with spiritual powers, using it to ward off evil spirits. Because of its strong smell, like its equally smelly relatives mint and oregano, it was used to relieve respiratory problems such as asthma, bronchitis and coughing.

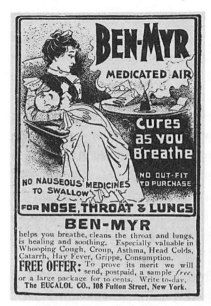
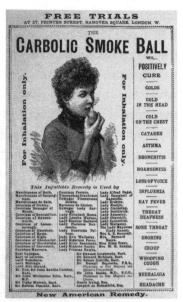

Ben Myr's medicated air 'cures as you breathe', and was advertised
in 1900 as being able to cure every known respiratory condition.
The active ingredient was eucalyptus oil.

Carbolic smoke ball claimed to cure a whole range of conditions associated
with breathing. The compressable ball was filled with phenol (carbolic acid),
and when squeezed the vapour would be released via the tube inserted
into a nostril. This noxious vapour would make the nose run vigorously,
supposedly flushing out any contaminants. The inventor,
one Mr Roe, died of TB aged 57 (handbill *c.* 1890).

Lungwort (*Pulmonaria officinalis*) is a small common garden
plant or herb from mainland Europe that does not emit any
noticeable vapours or alter breathing but is included in many
herbariums. The plant gets its common name from its white spotted leaves, which are suggestive of the lobular structure of the
lungs. Herbalists, who were the chief practitioners of folk medicine in the Middle Ages, considered that if a plant resembled a
body part it could cure disease associated with that body part. This
link between form and function dates back to Dioscorides and
Galen and was eventually formalized by the German herbalist and
theologian Jakob Boehme in his book *The Signature of All Things*
(1621), where the link of function and form was thought to be
God's signature, signposting the plant's usefulness to humankind.

Lungwort, with its spotted leaves, looked like a diseased lung. It was used to treat tuberculosis, asthma and coughs. Paracelsus (1493–1541) in his *Doctrine of Signatures* originally ascribed lungwort this function. Extracts of lungwort do work when used in a cough syrup, acting as an expectorant and clearing mucus. A further reflection of the doctrine of Paracelsus was practised by Sir Theodore Turquet de Mayerne (1573–1655), an influential Genevan physician who treated the nobility and royalty of Europe. When he moved to England he treated James I and his wife, Anne of Denmark, his main contribution to medicine was realizing the need to standardize medicine formulation. His cure for treating someone with breathing difficulties was 'a syrup made with the flesh of tortoises, snails and the lungs of animals, frogs, and crawfish (crayfish), all boiled in scabrous and coltsfoot water, adding at the last sugar candy, will prove very useful'. This mixture reflects the belief that a medicine made of animal lungs would overcome breathing problems.[36]

A lichen called tree lungwort (*Lobaria pulmonaria*) is often confused with the garden lungwort (*Pulmonaria officinalis*). It gets its name from its lobular structure, which resembles that of the lungs. Thus, following the *Doctrine of Signatures* by Paracelsus, the plant was used to treat respiratory ailments. The herbalist John Gerard in his book *The Herball; or, Generall Historie of Plants* (1597) recommends *Lobelia pulmonaria* as useful but it may be that the author was confused with lungwort.

Elecampane (*Inula helenium*) is a native of Europe and Asia and is a member of the sunflower family, an herbaceous plant with yellow flowers that look a bit like dandelions. The name 'helenium' is supposedly derived from Helen of Troy, as the plant is said to have sprouted from the ground where her tears fell during her captivity after her abduction by Paris. It was also called elfwort by the Celts, to whom it was sacred. The root contains the active ingredients, providing an expectorant that eases mucus flow in the airways and is still used today in herbal remedies.

Lobelia (*Lobelia inflata*) and osha root (*Ligusticum porteri*) are plants from North America that have been used for centuries

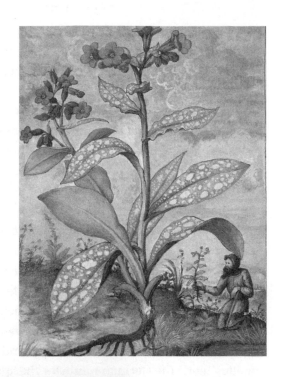

Two lungworts, the plant *Pulmonaria officinalis* and the lichen *Lobaria pulmonaria* (or tree lungwort), copied from nature and shown in their natural environment. Illustrations from Gherardo Cibo, *Dioscorides' de re Medica* (1564–84).

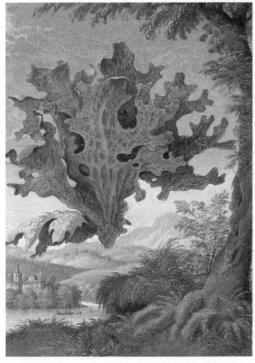

as medicinal remedies. Osha root was used by Native Americans as a medicine for a range of maladies and when used as a mouth-wash or tea it was taken for sore throats. In more recent times it has been used to treat tuberculosis. Osha root is said be a bron-chodilator, opening the airways and helping breathing. Lobelia leaves, when smoked or chewed, have many effects on the heart and act as a purgative. When given to someone with an asthma attack, they serves to relieve the symptoms. Its action is similar to a medical product called Asthmador, which, from the 1920s, was smoked in cigarette form by people with asthma. The active ingredient was the alkaloid hyoscyamine, contained in the plant belladonna or deadly nightshade (*Atropa belladonna*). These medicines were replaced by inhalers in the 1950s.

Asafoetida is a pungent-smelling powder derived from dried sap extracted from the stems and root of the plant *Ferula asafoe-tida*, a member of the celery family.[37] The etymology of *asafoetida* comes from the Persian for 'resin', *asa*, and the Latin *foetidus*: smelling fetid. The German name for the spice is *Stinkasant* or *Reufelsdreck* (stinking gum). The plant is a native to Central Asia, Iran and Afghanistan and has been known since ancient times. It still used today, giving Worcestershire sauce its distinct bitter flavour. Once ingested, it does not leave a smell on the breath, as onions or garlic do. Throughout history asafoetida has been used to treat many conditions, but it has been used widely as an expectorant to treat pneumonia, and asthma.

Yew (*Taxus baccata*) trees are one of the most ancient trees growing widely across the northern hemisphere. The ancient Greeks and Egyptians valued the yew's dark, heavy wood. Yew is not usually associated with breathing, but it has a close asso-ciation with causing and preventing death. Yew needles, bark and berries are all toxic and when ingested can be lethal, causing cardiogenic shock and respiratory failure. One of the early symp-toms of toxicity is rapid breathing and a feeling of breathlessness, which is then followed by the slowing of breathing until it stops. Those poisoned do not respond to attempts at artificial resuscita-tion. Even the pollen is toxic and exposure to the pollen can trigger asthma. In regions around the world where yew is common, yew extracts have been used to treat respiratory disorders. In Nepalese medicine the needles are used to treat coughs, bronchitis and asthma, while the Iroquois in North America use yew to treat coughs and colds.[38]

In medieval Europe and in particular in the UK, yew wood was found to be ideal for making longbows. Longbows were superior to bows made from other wood. Their superiority ensured that over the Middle Ages millions of these bows were made, leading to the virtual extinction of the yew in Europe. To draw a longbow requires plenty of strength and also for the archer to take a large breath in as they draw: this manoeuvre provides a feeling of power. Once the bow is fully drawn the breath is held and the target concentrated upon, and once met, the bowstring and arrow is released and the archer exhales, completely emptying the lungs. The longbow proved itself in many great battles:

Lott's Lung Pills of unknown composition, and another miracle cure for all known respiratory diseases, c. 1830s, handbill.

FOR THE CURE OF COUGHS, COLDS,
CONSUMPTION, ASTHMAS, &c.

LOTT'S
LUNG PILLS

have justly obtained the unqualified approbation of all those who have tried them for speedily curing the Influenza and Bronchitis; also as a most valuable and efficacious Remedy for Colds, Catarrhs, Coughs, Hoarseness, Difficulty of Breathing, Asthma, Consumption, Spitting of Blood; and all disorders of the Lungs. In violent and distressing Coughs they never fail to afford immediate relief, by allaying the tickling and irritation of the Throat and Windpipe, which is the cause of frequent Coughing. They promote Expectoration, remove Fever, Lassitude, and Chilliness. Public Orators and the most Celebrated Vocalists have long held them in the highest estimation for their invaluable properties in removing Huskiness, Wheezing, and Oppression of the Chest, Strengthening the Lungs, and giving Power, Tone, and Clearness to the Voice. A Dose at bed-time seldom fails to cure a recent Cold, and procure sound and refreshing Sleep.

Sold by Appointment of the Proprietor, by

J. W. STIRLING, CHEMIST,
86, HIGH STREET, WHITECHAPEL,
From whom a SINGLE DOSE can be had; or in Stamped Boxes at 18½d., 2s. 9d., 4s. 6d. & 11s. each.

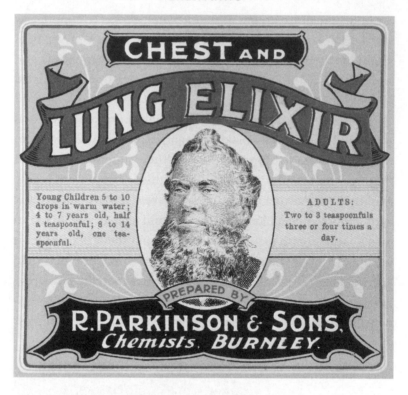

Victorian patent medicine trade card advertising Parkinson & Sons'
Chest and Lung Elixir, given to pharmacists to advertise manufacturer's
wares, *c.* 1900.

in 1346 at the Battle of Crécy, France, an estimated 7,000 English
longbow archers released around 70,000 arrows a minute, inflict-
ing heavy casualties on the French. Being on the receiving end of
these arrow storms was lethal, but the archers would have been
disciplined: breathe in, hold, release and exhale. It was synchro-
nized breathing on a large scale. By Tudor times yew wood for
bows was becoming hard to find, so Elizabeth I made muskets
the official weapon of choice.

The yew enters our story of breathing again in the 1960s when
Taxol, an extract from yew bark, was found to prevent cancers,
including lung cancer. Suddenly yew bark was in demand and
that demand continued to grow over the next few decades, ensuring that millions of trees were felled in North America and Asia,
areas that were not accessed in earlier times. Eventually the drug

was synthesized, using the needles as the starting material. Using needles is sustainable as it does not require the tree to be felled. Many yew plantations were created, saving the tree from near extinction a second time.[39]

THE CONNECTION BETWEEN breathing and emotion allows us to direct our breathing, giving us the ability to speak and sing. We can express our emotions through laughter in joyful moments and screaming when we face terror and fear. Emotions such as these, or conditions where we lose control of our breath, can lead to overbreathing and panic attacks. The main positive aspects to changing the way we breathe have been known for centuries, and breathing control is practised today in many ways. Yoga is one of the most popular forms, with millions of people welcoming the positive boost it provides to their mental health, mindfulness and well-being. The use of botanical extracts to aid breathing has contributed greatly to our health, but also to our understanding of how disease affects our breathing. Their impact has created a vast pharmaceutical industry, especially in treating the symptoms of the common cold, and with inhalers in the treatment of asthma and COPD.

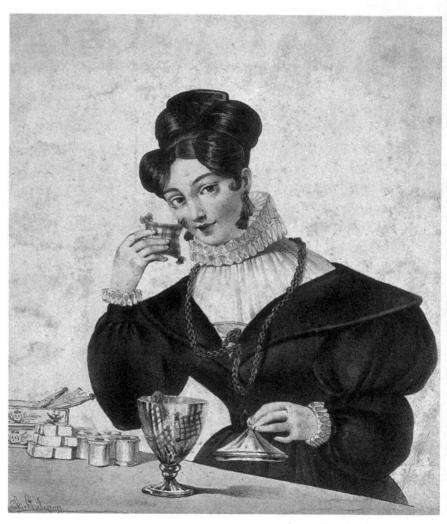

'The pleasant perfumer. A Paris perfume seller with a bag of lavender.
A popular French fragrance'. Illustration by Charles Philipon, 1828.

EIGHT

INSPIRED BREATHING

Breathing is such an ethereal and everyday occurrence that it is rarely the subject of poems, works of art, books or cultural phenomena. It does, however, feature in many English phrases and idioms. Before our modern understanding of breathing, early writers saw breathing in the context of pneuma, as a spiritual phenomenon. In fiction it was considered as a gentle breeze or as a spirit providing a vital life force. As we reach modern times, breathing becomes more visceral. Most modern works of fiction are permeated with a plethora of references to breathing, where it is used to signify heightened emotional states. Films with a breathing theme do exist and feature stories about extreme environments or the consequences of chronic respiratory disease.

There many phrases and idioms in the English language associated with breathing, be they physical, psychological or comical. One can talk 'under one's breath'. Less complimentary is the expression, 'I wouldn't breathe the same air' or the sarcastic retort 'pardon me for breathing,' which can be followed with 'what a waste of breath' (which is related to the more archaic saying about 'saving one's breath to cool one's porridge'). To have someone 'breathing down your neck' is not a pleasant experience, giving the sense of being overly pressurized by someone or something.

On a more positive note there are phrases such as 'like a breath of fresh air' or to 'take someone's breath away', usually referring to an inspiring or cheerful event. 'Catching one's breath' can signify the straightforward act of resting to overcome a temporary bout of breathlessness or can be uttered in order to initiate a brief pause to collect one's thoughts or plan ahead for what to do next. The phrases 'to breathe a sigh of relief', 'breathing room' and 'breathing space' all speak for themselves, as does 'take a breather'.

A common phrase is 'with bated breath', or sometimes the malapropism 'with baited breath', the title of a Warhammer novel by George Mann. This phrase is frequently used but has obscure origins. At first it may seem to imply that the subject has halitosis, but this is not the case. It was first used by Shakespeare in the comedy *The Merchant of Venice*, by the character Shylock:

> SHYLOCK: Shall I bend low, and in a servant's whine, with bated breath and whispering humbleness say, 'Sir you spit on me on Wednesday last.'

'Bated' is a short form of the word 'abated'. The phrase 'bated breath' was popular in Victorian times, especially in the numerous melodramatic novels popular at the time. Good illustrative examples can be found in the novels of Georg Ebers, the German Egyptologist who discovered the medical papyri that bear his name. Ebers tried to popularize his discoveries through writing historical romances. In his novel *A Thorny Path* from 1892, his characters 'listened with outstretched necks and bated breath', 'stood at the window with bated breath' and 'listened with bated breath'.

'Don't breathe a word' is a usually issued as a warning, asking someone to keep a secret. The opposite is found in 'long-winded', when a person speaks for an unnecessarily long time. Even inanimate items can breathe, such as wine, and in times gone by the medical practice of breathing a vein was considered good medicine and used to treat many a condition or illness.

The ancient Greeks, without our modern view of breathing, saw only pneuma and aether. Homer made effective use of these phenomena in his epic poems *The Odyssey* and *The Iliad*. In the first, *The Odyssey*, Homer equates peace and tranquillity with breathing, often referring to the gentle breath of the wind and evoking a quiet and peaceful climate: 'the gods becalmed me twenty days without so much as a breath of fair wind to help me forward', or 'Minerva took the form of the famous sea captain Dymas's daughter . . . then, coming up to the girl's bedside like a breath of wind, she hovered over her head.'

In stark contrast, in the more bloodthirsty *Iliad*, which includes the siege of Troy, where the Greeks battled the Trojans, the loss of breath or pneuma signifies the loss of life. Many warriors die in this epic, such as Achilles: 'Long as Achilles breathes this vital air' and 'The corpse now breathless on the bloody plain'. Furthermore, breathing is commonly attached to an emotion or behaviour: 'Breathing revenge, in arms they take their way' and 'Thus they, breathing united force with fixed thought, Moved on in silence.'

The fiction of Geoffrey Chaucer (1343–1400) includes the notion of pneuma, and its function as a vital life force and as a mechanism to cool the body, with the lungs considered the engine of the body.[1] In the *Canterbury Tales* the first tale, *The Knights Tale* (1386–8), explores the effects of love on two cousins, Palamon and Arcite, and ends with Arcite dying after being thrown from his horse. Here Chaucer describes the death in detail: after the heart stops beating, the 'pipes of his longes' 'shent with venym and corrupcioun'. In other words, the circulation of the blood ceases, and the lungs cannot cool the body anymore. The final demise happens thus: 'Dusked his eyen two and failled breeth' with the loss of breathing marking the point of death. This passage provides a good view of medical knowledge at the time, reflecting the view that breath was a vital life force.

Shakespeare's works contain many references to breathing, both dramatic and functional, such as in the following exchange from Romeo and Juliet:

> NURSE: Jesu, what haste! Can you not stay awhile? Do you not see that I am out of breath?
> JULIET: How art thou out of breath when thou hast breath to say to me that thou art out of breath? The excuse that thou dost make in this delay is longer than the tale thou dost excuse.' (II.5)

Shakespeare even offers a new technical term to describe breathing: 'suspiration'. 'Nor windy suspiration of forced breath, No, nor the fruitful river of the eye' (*Hamlet*, 1.2). This refers to a long deep sigh, the windy and forced component implying that the sigh is falsely generated.[2] It is a useful word, but one rarely used in modern language or at all in medicine. An example is given by T. S. Eliot, who after surviving bombing in the London Blitz in his poem 'Little Gidding' (1942) muses on being destroyed by the fires of war or the fire of the Holy Spirit. The fourth stanza of the poem begins: 'The dove descending breaks the air' and ends:

> The intolerable shirt of flame.
> Which Human power cannot remove.
> We only live, only suspire
> Consumed by either fire or fire.

Some people argue that Shakespeare wrote his lines in such a way that they were best delivered with a pause after each line and a breath taken before the next line. Today this is known as Hall's pause. This idea is controversial, as this might suit the actor in delivering their lines to a rhythm, but most audiences find it a distraction.

Sir Walter Scott (1771–1832) reflects the mechanistic view of breathing coming to the fore in his novel *The Fair Maid of Perth*: '"Then I am so accustomed to the use of arms, and so well breathed, that few men can match me" said the little man, expanding his breast . . . "here is room for all the wind machinery"'.

The English poet and playwright John Dryden (1631–1700) used breathing to dramatize death: 'In vain: if sword and poison be denied me, I'll hold my breath and die' and 'The youth though in haste, / And breathing his last, / In pity died slowly, while she died more fast'. In the next verse a nymph persuades a young shepherd to revive himself so that she can die slowly and he more quickly, a noble act.

A book which covers many of the early twentieth-century issues concerning the discovery of industrial lung disease and thought by some to have influenced the Welsh Labour Party politician Aneurin Bevan (1897–1960)in his views on the structure of the National Health Service in the UK was *The Citadel*, published in 1937 by A. J. Cronin, a Scottish-born doctor-turned-novelist.[3] It was an instant best-seller and in 1938 was made into the MGM film *Citadel*, starring Robert Donat and Rosalind Russell. The book follows the career of a newly qualified doctor, Andrew Manson, starting with his first job serving the coal-mining communities of the South Wales valleys as an inexperienced young doctor and ending with treating only wealthy private patients from his own practice in Central London. Apart from providing a commentary on medicine during the pre-NHS period, the book is notable because Manson is interested in pulmonary medicine. In the Welsh valleys he comes across miners with pneumoconiosis and tuberculosis. At the time coal dust was considered inert. Conducting research on the miners and later guinea pigs, he discovers the cause of the miners' lung disease, postulating that exposure to silica leads to tuberculosis. This is of course wrong: the author, Cronin, was unaware of pneumoconiosis. In the book Manson is expelled from his post in the Welsh valleys after his unlawful vivisection is discovered. In London he falls for the luxuries afforded by treating wealthy clients. He practises in the leading London Chest hospital but soon realizes that London is too foggy and polluted for TB patients. He advocates the ideas of the sanatorium in the cleaner airs of the home counties. The book closes with Dr Manson facing the General Medical Council for trying to cure TB by assisting in the deliberate creation of pneumothorax. The idea behind the treatment being that the collapsed lung would recuperate while resting and unventilated. This was a fashionable but illegal idea at the time and was later proved not to work. The doctor is cleared in the end. Cronin went on to create the 1960s television series *Dr Finlay's Casebook*.

Modern fiction writers show a good knowledge of the mechanism of breathing and its relationship to emotion and behaviour. An example can be found in the first chapter of *Broken Ground*, published by Val McDermid in 2018. It opens in 1944 in Wester

Ross, Scotland, where two men are digging pits. 'The slaps of spades in dense peat was an unmistakable sound. They slipped in and out of rhythm; overlapping, separating, cascading, then coming together again, much like the men's heavy breathing.' Later, one rests with his 'breath tight in his chest'. After a night of hard toil, their task is complete, and the chapter ends with the line: 'Even as he spoke, the *Mycobacterium tuberculosis* organisms were creeping through his lungs, destroying tissues, carving out holes, blocking airways.' The character dies of TB, setting the scene for the story firmly set in the twenty-first century.

In Jo Nesbo's detective novel *Knife* (2019), the leading character, Harry Hole, is about to hear from the police unwelcome news about his partner Rakel: 'Harry held his breath. He had read that it was possible to hold your breath for so long that you died. And that you don't die from too little oxygen, but from too much carbon dioxide.' When told that they have found her, he wanted to ask why and thought to himself 'But to do that [I] would have to breathe.' He breathed. 'And that means "what?", he asked. "She's dead, Harry".'

Perfume: The Story of a Murderer (1985) is a tour de force of the olfactory sense, breathing and the craft of perfumery, written by the German author Patrick Süskind. The main character is Jean-Baptiste Grenouille, born in 1738, abandoned by his mother at birth, brought up by the Church and fostered by wet-nurses and childminders. Born without an odour, he soon realizes in his childhood that he has a superhuman sense of smell and can identify not only very subtle smells but the components of the odour. The book begins in Paris, a crowded and very smelly city. He starts life working for a tanner, a very smelly occupation. He secures an apprenticeship with an aged perfumer who has fallen on hard times, lacking a new perfume with which to entice his rich clients. With some scepticism from his employer, Grenouille is given access to the perfumer's collection of chemicals and scents and in a few days produces dozens of new perfumes which are so popular that they are soon produced on an industrial scale and sold all over Europe, making the perfumer a wealthy man.

The book illustrates how we take our sense of smell for granted and how we are surrounded by many familiar smells. Breathing and olfaction sets our emotions and behaviours: the invigorating smell of freshly brewed coffee in the morning, the smell of freshly baked bread stimulating hunger. Breathing the fragrance of fresh mown grass brings back memories of a summer long past. We recognize the scent of our loved ones, of babies and pets. These scents are all different, but we learn to enjoy or detest them.

After leaving Paris, Grenouille gains his credentials as a perfumer and sets off to Grasse in southern France to learn more about creating scents from flowers and plants. On his journey he invents a series of personal perfumes, which he cynically uses to influences people's opinion of him. One allows him to be the centre of attention, with everyone treating him like a celebrity; another keeps everyone away. They are scents that alter people's behaviour without the beholder noticing; something all modern scent manufacturers wish to do nowadays. Many of today's perfume- or fragrance-makers employ adverts to indicate that your attractiveness will be increased if you wear their fragrance.

On his journey south, at Montpellier, Grenouille meets the Marquis de la Taillade-Espinasse, a man influenced by the Enlightenment who has developed the idea that the earth generates a toxic gas which he calls Fluidium letale Taillade. Grenouille, who is looking rough after living in a cave for seven years, provides the marquis with a perfect example of the ill-effects of this terrestrial gas. His reasoning is that all living things move upwards away from the ground to avoid this gas. To test this theory, the marquis has invented a vital ventilation machine in his cellar, inside which Grenouille is sealed. The breathing machine is constantly ventilated with air drawn from a flue extended out of the house roof. Through an air-lock he is fed food from 'earth-removed' regions such as dove bouillon, lark pie and fruit picked from trees. The total recovery of Grenouille following this treatment proves to the marquis that his theory was correct. With this in mind the marquis departs on an expedition to the Pic du Canigou, in the French Pyrenees, which can be snow-capped for most of the year. The

Marquis believes that living at altitude will make him superhuman by being free from the evil Fludium latale, the cause of all illness. The marquis is last seen ascending the mountain. Pic du Canigou was also visited by Sir Humphry Davy in January 1814, who was so impressed by its natural form and light that it inspired him to sketch the mountain and write a poem, 'The Canigou', which alludes to the geological forces of nature.

The portrayal of breathing is significant in some films. One of the most famous film characters known for their breathing is Darth Vader from the *Star Wars* films. In his youth, in his former life as Anakin Skywalker, Vader is severely burned, after which he can only breath through a full-face mask (rather like a motorcycle helmet). The mask gives his slow, steady breathing a very distinctive mechanical and sinister sound. Mask breathing also features in the psychological thriller *Blue Velvet* (1986). Here the character Frank Booth, played by Dennis Hopper, carries two cylinders of gas, which he breathes through a mask. These allow him to change his personality, swapping between 'Daddy' and 'Baby'. The original idea was that the gas was helium, and when breathed it would raise the adult voice so that the character would sound like a child. In the end the gas is more 'pharmacological' than this and may act more like amyl nitrite.

Breathing is a common motif in films, not overtly, but in a subtle way, and is common in certain genres such as horror, melodrama and pornography. Here screaming, panting and hyperventilation are used to impart mood and promote the impact of the drama. Studies have shown that in general the emphasis of breathing on-screen is off-putting for the audience and is best left under the radar of perception and cognition. Thus the sound of breathing or lack of it is a conscious omission from many films and TV programmes. As one researcher states, 'no one is ever just breathing.'[4]

While smoking is often depicted in films, there are few feature films that focus on respiratory disease. A recent example is the film *Breathe* (2017), a biographical drama about Robin Cavendish, who while living in Kenya in 1958 caught polio at the age of 28, having just married. He became paralysed from the neck down and could only breathe with a bedside respirator. After returning to the UK he was bedridden and given only a few months to live. After the birth of his son raised his spirits, he set about improving his quality of life by improving his bedside ventilator. The film illustrates his long struggle to convince his doctors and the medical profession that his improved ventilator, when incorporated into a wheelchair, is a great advance over the iron lung then used by many doctors to keep paralysed polio patients alive. His ventilator was so mobile that it allowed him to travel abroad and live a fuller life. It is an inspiring story with a tragic ending, as eventually the many years of mechanical ventilation fatally destroyed his lungs. He died at the age of 64, one of the longest surviving responauts, as they are called.

The film *Apollo 13* (1995) tells the true story of the survival of the astronauts of the NASA mission in 1970. Tragedy struck two days in as an oxygen tank exploded in the service module. Fortunately, this was not the only supply of oxygen, but the mission had to be abandoned and the astronauts returned to Earth by using a slingshot circumnavigation of the moon to propel the crew back to Earth just before their oxygen ran out and the carbon dioxide levels in the cabin became toxic. The astronauts all returned safely to breathe another day. *Last Breath* (2019), a remarkable film in documentary style, details the true story of a deep-sea diver who while repairing an oil installation on the bottom of the North Sea is suddenly left without an oxygen supply. On the surface the support ship loses its position over the divers owing to a stormy sea, and the umbilical cord connected to the diver via a diving bell lowered from the ship and providing him with heat, air and power becomes tangled around an underwater installation and snaps. The diver is left with a small rescue tank carried for such emergencies that only contains 5 minutes of air. With the ship moving, the refuge of the diving bell also moves away, leaving the diver alone on the bottom of the North Sea. The sea is so rough that the crew struggle to return the ship to its original position, eventually taking around 30 minutes. When the ship's main cameras refocus on the diver, he is lying motionless on top of the structure. His diving buddy, who had made it safely back to the diving bell before the ship had lost position, was tasked with recovering the body and bringing it back to the diving bell. Once inside the diving bell, the recovered diver is given mouth-to-mouth resuscitation, and to everyone's surprise he instantly comes back to life. After a few months, the diver recovered completely. It is thought that he survived so long without oxygen as his body was cooled and super-saturated with oxygen: he had spent a long time in a hyperbaric chamber before the dive.

The film *The Aeronauts* (2019) is a biographical adventure film about two balloonists, a scientist and a professional balloonist (based on Sophie Blanchard, the wife of the balloonist Jean-Pierre Blanchard) in the 1800s who attempt to explore the upper atmosphere, with disastrous consequences.

THE ENGLISH LANGUAGE is rich with phrases involving the act of breathing, both mechanically and sensually. Literature has used this rich source to express and emphasize the drama and pathos of many works, from ancient times, through Shakespeare, to modern times. It is through the depiction of disaster, disease and adversity that we are told the consequences of not being able to breathe. In literature the boundary between life and death is often signified by the presence or absence of breathing and it is in the final chapter that we explore how we make one final great gesture before we pass away: our last breath.

NINE

LAST GASP

B reathing is a vital sign of life, continuous and relentless. One day it ceases. Cessation marks the end of life, or at the very least the final approach of death. The end is often witnessed and marked by the last breath, which is often the only physical sign of life, especially if the dying person is asleep or unconscious. This final breath can be quiet and imperceptible or dramatic and pronounced. It is often referred to as the last gasp, or, even more grandly, as the death rattle. The last breath may even be used to utter a few final words. Sometimes the final gasp is a peaceful one, sometimes it is troubled. In *Romeo and Juliet* Shakespeare wrote: 'Death, that hath suck'd the honey of thy breath, Hath had no power yet upon thy beauty' (Act v, Scene iii).

When a person is found unconscious lying on the floor, we apply ABC: airways, breathing and circulation. Once the person is positioned correctly, providing an open airway, palpation of the person's pulse is essential to see if the person's heart is pumping. CPR and mouth-to-mouth resuscitation can restore breathing and blood circulation. Failure to restore breathing marks death. The vital spark of life leaves the body as no more oxygen is consumed or carbon dioxide produced. Without blood flow and ventilated lungs, the movement of oxygen stops. Being asleep is a similar state to being unconscious, so if a person's life ends while they are asleep, breathing can simply fade away, slowly getting shallower and slower until eventually it stops, or ending with a sudden stutter or gasp.

The noisiest way to breathe one's last is the death rattle. This is thought to be caused by the accumulation of mucus and fluid in the lungs and throat as swallowing becomes difficult. The resulting gasping and laboured breath are known as agonal breathing or respiration. While it is unpleasant for the dying person, it is also very distressing for those attending the death. It can last just a few breaths or for several hours.

In literature the death rattle is used to provide dramatic focus. In Gustave Flaubert's novel *Madame Bovary* of 1856, the heroine, Emma Bovary, dies a tortured death:

> Her breast began rising and falling in rapid gasps. Her tongue protruded from her mouth. She would have been considered dead if it had not been for the terrifying movements of her ribs, faster and faster, driven by her desperate breathing, as if the soul was struggling violently to break free.

As everyone surrounded her deathbed, 'as the death-rattle grew more pronounced, the priest prayed faster'. Emma makes a final dramatic rally before dying. The chapter ends with the words 'She no longer existed.' Flaubert was able to give such a detailed dramatic description through quizzing his father and brother, who were both doctors and between them had experienced many final moments.

Similarly, the Russian writer Leo Tolstoy, in his 1886 novella *The Death of Ivan Ilych*, wrote about a high court judge's illness and his final prolonged death. 'For those present his agony continued for another two hours. Something rattled in his chest; his emaciated body twitched. Then rattling and wheezing gradually diminished,' and death occurred.

These dramatic fictional accounts of the final moments of death reflect reality. Many have died of respiratory diseases that today are curable, such as TB. Benjamin Franklin died from pleurisy at home in 1790, aged 84. Towards the end of his illness he was bedbound and in great pain, as breathing was difficult. One day his breathing was no longer painful. The family were pleased and thought he was better, but later in the day a cyst burst in his lungs and discharged a purulent matter, which made Franklin vomit. After this, his breathing gradually quietened as his lungs failed, and he died a few hours later at 11 p.m.

Death and breathing are intimately linked, marking the boundary between this life and the next. With advances in medical technology, the definition of death as stopping when breathing does is no longer valid, as breathing can be supported or maintained using mechanical ventilation. For example, people with bulbar poliomyelitis cannot breathe unassisted (because of brain stem damage), but when given mechanical ventilation can live for many decades. It was during the end of the nineteenth century that the first evidence emerged that certified death through either apnoea (lack of breathing) or asystole (lack of a pulse, circulatory or cardiac death) alone was insufficient, and that 'nervous system death or 'neurological death' was a more precise marker of death. Today this condition is known as brain death, or brain-stem death.

People who receive a severe head trauma, suffer a brain abscess or experience large intracranial bleeds can die of apnoea. Their breathing stops, quickly followed by their heart, as the supply of oxygenated blood ceases. One common feature of trauma is raised fluid pressure in the skull. It is this increase in pressure that stops the breathing. Our brains are bathed in a carefully regulated volume of fluid (the intracranial cerebral fluid, ICF). The ICF volume is small, as the space between the brain and skull is compact. Trauma results in the production of extra ICF fluid, which has nowhere to go, raising the intracranial pressure. The raised pressure compresses the brain tissues. At the base of the skull there is a hole through which the spinal cord connects with the projecting brain stem. The raised pressure causes the brain stem to become compressed from the bulk of the brain above. Eventually, if left untreated, it damages the respiratory centre and breathing stops and death occurs. The heart continues to beat for as long as oxygen is present, because it has its own built-in pacemaker, provided by the sinoatrial node, and can beat independently of the brain stem.

Of course, this was unknown in the nineteenth century. The first clinical reports appeared in 1892, when the English surgeon W. H. Jalland noted that breathing returned when pus was removed from an infected ear. In this case the removal of the pus had relieved the raised intracranial pressure. These observations were expanded by Victor Horsley, a London surgeon who in 1894 stated that patients with cerebral haemorrhage, brain tumours and depressed fractures of the skull 'die from respiratory and not cardiac failure'. Finally, the link between raised intracranial pressure and respiratory failure was made by the American neurosurgeon Harvey Cushing, who in 1902 stated that cardiac death was preceded by death of the brain stem and the respiratory centre. This suggested a cure by surgical intervention: the skull could be trepanned and the pressure relieved by draining the excess cerebrospinal fluid (CSF), the fluid surrounding the brain.

At this point death was still thought to be due to apnoea. This view changed after it became possible to directly measure brain activity. This was first achieved in 1924 by the German psychiatrist Hans Berger (1873–1941) using his invention the electroencephalogram machine or EEG. Berger discovered in the human brain what today we call the alpha wave rhythm, but which he named the 'Berger Wave' after himself.[1] Although he is known as the father of the EEG he later helped the Third Reich promote eugenics, leading to enforced sterilization of 400,000 young adults from 1933 onwards, compared to 30,000 in the USA. By 1945 these unfortunate people were deemed 'life unworthy of life' and 275,000 were killed.[2]

When the EEG signal disappears the brain could be said to be dead, even though (supported) breathing and the heart and all other body functions continue as normal. The brainless body can be supported via liquid feeding nutrition and hydration. In 1959 the term 'coma dépassé' was coined to describe the condition by two leading clinicians in the field. It was not until 1968 that a person with brain-stem death was deemed dead. This is different from comatose, when breathing can be unsupported and brain-stem damage is minimal.

With the improvements in paramedicine, ambulance transport, emergency medicine and the establishment of the intensive care unit, those receiving brain injuries can be treated before the intracranial pressure becomes lethal and their breathing supported with mechanical ventilation throughout, keeping the heart and brain supplied with oxygen and allowing the heart and brain to stay healthy. This treatment buys the person time to recover. Any intracranial blood clot can be broken up and blood flow to the brain restored, allowing the intracranial pressure to be restored and the patient to make a full recovery. However, in some cases the intracranial pressure can be so great that blood flow to the brain ceases altogether. When this happens, the brain dies but the heart and lungs remain healthy; this person is irreversibly unconscious (dead) but with a body that is able to function, a condition unknown before the invention of mechanical ventilation. This has opened up a completely new area of medicine: organ transplantation. Keeping the body's organs alive by mechanical ventilation allows surgeons to carefully remove them for use in others who need them. Kidneys, livers and hearts can be transplanted in this way. Even the lungs can be transplanted; typically the recipient is a young person with cystic fibrosis.[3]

To the ancient Egyptians death was not the end, so they prepared their dead for an afterlife, and so were concerned that they should be able to breathe, eat and drink there. The Pyramid texts, religious texts from the Old Kingdom (2400–2300 BC), describe a ceremony of the 'opening of the mouth' performed by priests to enable life after death. To the Sumerians, Babylonians and Assyrians, breathing and life were synonymous, and once breathing stopped life was over. They believed that humans were first created by the mixing of blood of a slain deity called We-ilu with clay, which gave humans an organic and spiritual component. Thus when breathing ceased the person was physically dead but considered asleep (the spiritual component); it was upon burial that the body turned back to clay (the organic component). Although the person was physically dead, their spiritual side lived on like a ghost, and was termed *gidim*. The *gidim* represented the personality of the person and transported them to their place in the netherworld, a shadowy and dull representation of earth.

The idea of bodies consisting of an earthly organic component and a spiritual component is found in the Christian Bible. God states, 'you are dust and to dust you shall return' (Genesis 3:19). Again, the spirit or soul lives on, waiting for resurrection, evidence of the soul's presence being their breathing. 'Pairs of all creatures that have the breath of life in them came to Noah' (Genesis 7:15).

In Hinduism, breathing is an essential attribute of the living, and absence of breath (*prana*) and breathing (*an*) signify death. Again, this is merely an organic death, as the soul (*atman*) remains and eternally joins the cosmos.

THE BEGINNING AND end of life are intimately associated with breathing: a large breath in, a cry, providing the first breath, and a gasp, breathing out, the last. In between there are hundreds of millions more breaths. We breathe slowly while we are asleep and faster when we exercise. Those of us who are fortunate enough to avoid lung disease and prolonged exposure to air pollution continue breathing unimpeded. Along the way emotion alters our breathing, the laughter of happy moments altering the rhythm; while we exercise our talents of singing, we train our breathing to enhance our voice. The history of our understanding of breathing is long and has exercised some of the greatest minds. Some have got it wrong; others faced death and adversity to find out more. Their small steps of discovery have led to breathing being understood in its myriad of variations, giving us the greatest opera singers, politicians and orators. Yet death from respiratory disease is set to be the greatest cause of death globally as tobacco smoking reaches epidemic proportions in Asia and air pollution is present in all the major cities of the world. Breathing, then, is the foremost of all our vital signs, central to a healthy life and continued well-being. Breathing is life, and life is breathing.

REFERENCES

ONE: THE BREATH OF LIFE

1 Donald E. Canfield, *Oxygen: A Four Billion Year History* (Princeton, NJ, 2014), pp. 196, 156.
2 Connie C. W. Hsia et al., 'Evolution of Air Breathing: Oxygen Homeostasis and the Transitions from Water to Land and Sky', *Comparative Physiology*, III (2013), pp. 849–915.
3 Sarah K. Griffiths and Jeremy P. Campbell, 'Placental Structure, Function and Drug Transfer', *Continuing Education in Anaesthesia, Critical Care and Pain*, XV (2015), pp. 84–9.
4 J. G. Nijhuis et al., 'The Rhythmicity of Fetal Breathing Varies with Behavioural State in the Human Fetus', *Early Human Development*, IX (1983), pp. 1–7.
5 Peter Lewis and Peter Boylan, 'Fetal Breathing: A Review', *American Journal of Obstetrics and Gynaecology*, CXXXIV (1979), pp. 587–98.
6 Ibid.
7 M. Obladen, '*Pulmo Uterinus:* A History of Ideas on Fetal Respiration', *Journal of Perinatal Medicine*, XLI (2018), pp. 457–64.
8 John Bostock, *An Elementary System of Physiology*, vol. II (London, 1826), p. 643.
9 S. Joshi et al., 'Exercise-induced Bronchoconstriction in School-aged Children Who Had Chronic Lung Disease in Infancy', *Journal of Pediatrics*, CLXII (2013), pp. 813–18.
10 Rhea Urs et al., 'Persistent and Progressive Long-term Lung Disease in Survivors of Preterm Birth', *Paediatric Respiratory Reviews*, XXVI (2018), pp. 87–94.

TWO: EARLY BELIEFS

1 J. Kappelman et al., 'First Homo Erectus From Turkey and Implications for Migration Into Temperate Eurasia', *American Journal of Physical Anthropology*, CXXXV (2008), pp. 110–16.

2 Jakub Kwiecinski, 'Images of the Respiratory System in Ancient Egypt: Trachea, Bronchi and Pulmonary Lobes', *Canadian Respiratory Journal*, XIX (2012) pp. 33–4.

3 Ibid.

4 Friedrich Solmsen, 'The Vital Heat, the Inborn Pneuma and the Aether', *Journal of Hellenic Studies*, LXXVII (1957), pp. 119–23.

5 Ernest Best, 'The Use and Non-use of Pneuma by Josephus', *Novum Testamentum*, III (1959), pp. 218–25.

6 Kishor Patwardhan, 'The History of the Discovery of Blood Circulation: Unrecognized Contributions of Ayurveda Masters', *Advances in Physiology Education*, XXXVI (2012), pp. 77–82.

7 Aparna Singh, 'Physiological Appraisal of Prana Vayu in Ayurvedic Literatures', *International Journal of Physiology, Nutrition and Physical Education*, III (2018), pp. 2157–9.

8 Pedzisai Mazengenya and Rashid Bhikha, 'An Analysis of Historical Vignettes by Ibn Sina in the Canon of Medicine on the Structure and Function of the Cardiorespiratory Apparatus', *Archives of Iranian Medicine*, XX (2017), pp. 386–8.

9 Seyyed Mehdi Hashemi and Mohsin Raza, 'The Traditional Diagnosis and Treatment of Respiratory Diseases: A Description From Avicenna's Canon of Medicine', *Therapeutic Advances in Respiratory Disease*, III (2009), pp. 319–28; John B. West, 'Ibn Al-Nafis, the Pulmonary Circulation, and the Islamic Golden Age', *Journal of Applied Physiology*, CV (2008), pp. 1877–80.

10 Reinaldo Bulgarelli Bestetti et al., 'Development of Anatomophysiologic Knowledge Regarding the Cardiovascular System: From Egypt to Harvey', *Arquivos Brasileiros de Cardiologia*, CIII (2014), 38S–45S.

11 Bryan Gandevia, 'The Breath of Life: An Essay on the Earliest History of Respiration. Part 1', *Australian Journal of Physiotherapy*, XVI (1970), pp. 5–11.

12 John W. Severinghaus, 'Eight Sages over Five Centuries Share Oxygen's Discovery', *Advances in Physiology Education*, XL (2016), pp. 370–76.

13 Concealed lung anatomy in Botticelli's masterpieces *The Primavera* and the *Birth of Venus*. Davide Lazzeri, *Acta Biomedica*, LXXXVIII, (2017), pp. 502–9.

14 Donald Fleming, 'Galen on the Motions of the Blood in the Heart and Lungs', *Isis*, XLVI (1955), pp. 14–21; Donald Fleming, 'William Harvey and the Pulmonary Circulation', *Isis*, XLVI (1955), pp. 319–27.

15 Leonard G. Wilson, 'The Transformation of Ancient Concepts of Respiration in the Seventeenth Century', *Isis*, LI (1960), pp. 161–72.

16 Lavoisier Antoine Laurent, *Encyclopaedia Britannica* (1971), vol. XIII, pp. 818–19.

17 M. J. Eadie, 'Robert Whytt and the Pupils', *Journal of Clinical Neuroscience*, VII (2000), pp. 295–7.

18 Charles F. Bolton et al., *Neurology of Breathing* (New York, 2004), pp. 3–18.

19 Tobias Cheung, 'Limits of Life and Death: Legallios's Decapitation Experiments', *Journal of the History of Biology*, XLVI (2013), pp. 283–313.

20 J.M.S. Pearce, 'Marie-Jean-Pierre Flourens (1794–1867) and Cortical Localization', *European Neurology*, CXI (2009), pp. 311–14.

21 D. Doyle, 'Eponymous Doctors Associated With Edinburgh, Part 2 – David Bruno, John Cheyne, William Stokes, Alexander Munro *Secundus*, Joseph Gamgee', *Journal of the Royal College of Physicians of Edinburgh*, XXVI (2006), pp. 374–81.

22 *New Scientist*, 15 July 1976, p. 160.

23 Ernest H. Starling, *Principles of Human Physiology*, 3rd edn (London, 1920), p. 1123.

24 Ibid.

25 Martin Fronius, Wolfgang G. Clauss and Mike Althaus, 'Why Do We Have to Move Fluid to Be Able to Breathe?', *Frontiers in Physiology*, III (2012), Article 146, pp. 1–9.

26 Klaus D. Jürgens et al., 'Heart and Respiratory Rates and Their Significance for Convective Oxygen Transport Rates in the Smallest Mammal, the Etruscan Shrew *Suncus etruscus*', *Journal of Experimental Biology*, CXCIX (1996), pp. 2579–84.

27 Andreas Fahlman, Michael J. Moore and Daniel Garcia-Parraga, 'Respiratory Function and Mechanics in Pinnipeds and Cetaceans', *Journal of Experimental Biology*, CCXX (2017), pp. 1761–73.

28 Toshio Kuroki, 'Physiological Essay on Gulliver's Travels: A Correction after Three Centuries', *Journal of Physiological Sciences*, LXIX (2019), pp. 421–4.

29 George Pearson, 'On the Colouring Matter of the Black Bronchial Glands and of the Black Spots of the Lungs', *Philosophical Transactions of the Royal Society, London*, XII (1813), pp. 159–70.

30 Charles A. Culotta, 'Respiration and Lavoisier Tradition: Theory and Modification, 1777–1850', *Transactions of the American Philosophical Society*, LXII (1972), pp. 3–41.

31 G. Valentin, *A Text Book of Physiology* (London, 1853).

32 W. Allen and W. H. Pepys, 'On the Changes Produced in Atmospheric Air and Oxygen Gas by Respiration', *Philosophical Transactions of the Royal Society, London*, XVII (1808), pp. 249–81.

THREE: **INDUSTRY AND REVOLUTION**

1 Lundy Braun, *Breathing Race into the Machine: The Surprising Career of Spirometer from Plantation to Genetics* (Minneapolis, MN, 2014), p. 271.

2 Heidi L Lujan and Stephen E. DiCarlo, 'Science Reflects History as Society Influences Science: Brief History of "Race", "Race Correction" and the Spirometer', *Advances in Physiology Education*, XLII (2018), pp. 163–5.

3 Ibid.

4 J. Cleeland and S. Burt, 'Charles Turner Thackrah: A Pioneer in the Field of Occupational Health', *Occupational Medicine*, XLV (1995), pp. 285–97.

5 Ibid.

6 Ibid.

7 John Hutchinson, 'Contributions to Vital Statistics, Obtained by Means of a Pneumatic Apparatus for Valuing the Respiratory Powers With Relation to Health', *Journal of the Statistical Society of London*, VII (1844), pp. 193–212.

8 Thomas L. Petty, 'John Hutchinson's Mysterious Machine Revisited', *Chest*, CXXI (2002), 219S–223S.

9 John Hutchinson, 'On the Capacity of the Lungs, and on the Respiratory Functions with a View of Establishing a Precise and Easy Method of Detection of Detecting Disease by the Spirometer', *Medico-Chirurgical Transactions*, XXIX (1846), pp. 137–252.

10 Edward J. Wood, *Giants and Dwarfs* (London, 1868), p. 497.

11 Petty, 'John Hutchinson's Mysterious Machine Revisited'.

12 Bryan Gandevia, 'John Hutchinson in Australia and Fiji', *Medical History*, XXI (1977), pp. 365–83.

13 Braun, *Breathing Race into the Machine*, p. 271.

14 Charles Gayarré, 'The Southern Question', *North American Review*, CXXV (1877), pp. 472–98.

15 Braun, *Breathing Race into the Machine*, p. 271.

16 *Quain's Dictionary of Medicine*, ed. H. Montague Murray (London, 1902), pp. 1228–39.

17 Sultan Ahmed et al., 'Host-directed Therapy as a Novel Treatment Strategy to Overcome Tuberculosis: Targeting Immune Modulation', *Antibiotics*, VIII (2019), pp. 1–19.

18 R. Tait McKenzie, *Exercise in Education and Medicine* (Philadelphia, PA, 1917), p. 585.

19 Ibid.

20 Braun, *Breathing Race into the Machine*, p. 271.

21 Ibid.

22 Weston Thatcher Borden et al., 'Dioxygen: What Makes This Triplet Diradical Kinetically Persistant', *Journal of the American Chemical Society*, CXXXIX (2017), pp. 9010–18.

23 John B. West, 'Three Classical Papers in Respiratory Physiology by Christian Bohr (1855–1911), Whose Work Is Frequently Cited But Seldom Read', *American Journal of Physiology – Lung Cell Molecular Physiology*, CCCXVI (2019), L585–L588.

24 C. Bohr, 'Über die spezifische Tätigkeit der Lungen bei der respiratorischen Gasaufnahme und ihr Verhalten zu der Durch die alveolarwand statt-findenden Gasdiffusion', *Skand Arch Physiol.*, XXII (1909), pp. 221–80.

25 Albert Gjedde, 'Diffusive Insights: On the Disagreement of Christian Bohr and August Krogh at the Centennial of the Seven Little Devils', *Advances in Physiology Education*, XXIV (2010), pp. 174–85.

26 A. Krogh and M. Krogh, 'On the Tensions of Gases in Arterial Blood', *Skandinavisches Archiv für Physiologie*, XXIII (1910), pp. 179–92; M. Krogh, 'The Diffusion of Gases Through the Lungs of Man', *Journal of Physiology*, XCIX (1915), pp. 271–300.

27 John T. Edsall, 'Blood and Haemoglobin: The Evolution of Knowledge of Functional Adaption in a Biochemical System. Part 1: The Adaptation of Chemical Structure to Function in Haemoglobin', *Journal of the History of Biology*, V (1972), pp. 205–57; John T. Edsall, 'Understanding Blood and Hemoglobin: An Example of International Relations in Science', *Perspectives in Biology and Medicine*, XXIX (1986), 107S–123S.

28 G. G. Stokes, 'On the Reduction and Oxidation of the Colouring Matter of the Blood', *Proceedings of the Royal Society of London*, XIII (1864), p. 355.

FOUR: MIASMA AND BAD AIR

1 Jacques Jouanna, 'Air, Miasma and Contagion in the Time of Hippocrates and the Survival of Miasmas in Post-Hippocratic Medicine (Rufus of Ephesus, Galen and Palladius)', in *Greek Medicine from Hippocrates to Galen* (Leiden, 2012), pp. 119–36.

2 Ibid.

3 Ibid.

4 J. T. Carter, 'Vitiated Air: A Victorian Villain?', *Journal of the Royal Society of Medicine*, LXXIV (1981), pp. 914–19.

5 M. J. Dobson, 'History of Malaria', *Journal of the Royal Society of Medicine*, Supplement 17, LXXXII (1989), pp. 3–7.

6 Richard Jones, *Mosquito* (London, 2012), p. 216.

7   Jun-Fang Sun, 'Medical Implication in the Bible and Its Relevance
    to Modern Medicine', *Journal of Integrative Medicine*, XI (2013),
    pp. 416–21.
8   Catharine Arnold, *Pandemic 1918: The Story of the Deadliest
    Influenza in History* (London, 2018), p. 357.
9   Ibid.
10 Alan W. Hampson, 'Avian Influenza: A Pandemic Waiting in the
    Wings?', *Emergency Medicine Australasia*, XVIII (2006), pp. 420–29;
    Jessica A. Belsar et al., 'Complexities in Ferret Influenza Virus
    Pathogenesis and Transmission Models', *Microbiology and
    Molecular Biology Reviews*, CXXX (2016), pp. 733–44.
11 Hampson, 'Avian Influenza', pp. 420–29.
12 Arnold, *Pandemic 1918*, p. 357.
13 Robert Harris and Jeremy Paxman, *A Higher Form of Killing: The
    Secret History of Chemical and Biological Warfare* (London, 2002),
    p. 300.
15 Ibid.
16 Ibid.
17 Ibid.
18 Peter J. Baxter, M. Kapila and D. Mfonfu, 'Lake Nyos Disaster,
    Cameroon, 1986: The Medical Effects of Large Scale Emission
    of Carbon Dioxide?', *British Medical Journal*, CCXCVIII (1989),
    pp. 1437–41.
19 Mark Miodownik, *Liquid Rules: The Delightful and Dangerous
    Substances That Flow Through Our Lives* (London, 2018), p. 276.
20 M. E. Jonasson and R. Afshari, 'Historical Documentation of Lead
    Toxicity Prior to the 20th Century in English Literature', *Human
    and Experimental Toxicology*, XXXVIII (2017), pp. 775–88.
21 Kassia St Clair, *The Secret Lives of Colour* (London, 2016), p. 43.
22 Philiberto Vernatti, 'A Relation of the Making of Ceruss by Sir
    Philiberto Vernatti', *Philosophical Transactions of the Royal
    Society of London*, XXXVII/12 (1677), pp. 935–6.
23 Kanta Sircar et al., 'Carbon Monoxide Poisoning Deaths in the
    United States, 1999 to 2012', *American Journal of Emergency
    Medicine*, XXXIII (2015), pp. 1140–45.
24 Hunter H. Comly, 'Cyanosis in Infants Caused by Nitrates in Well
    Water', *Journal of the American Medical Association*, CXXIX (1945),
    pp. 112–16.
25 Roger P. Smith, 'What Makes My Baby Blue', *Dartmouth Medicine*
    (Summer 2000), pp. 26–31, 51.
26 A. A. Avery, 'Infantile Methemoglobinemia: Re-examining
    the Role of Drinking Water Nitrates', *Environmental Health
    Perspectives*, CVII (1999), pp. 583–6; Alyce M. Richard, James H.

Diaz and Alan David Kaye, 'Re-examining the Risks of Drinking-water Nitrates on Public Health', *Ochsner Journal*, XIV (2014), pp. 392–8.

27 Arthur Musk et al., 'The Wittenoom Legacy', *International Journal of Epidemiology* (2019), pp. 1–10.

28 J. Robertson Wallace, *The Constitution of Man: Man in Health, Man in Disease*, 4th edn (London, 1897), p. 420.

29 Carter, 'Vitiated Air', pp. 914–19.

30 Eleanor Herman, *The Royal Art of Poison: Filthy Palaces, Fatal Cosmetics, Deadly Medicine and Murder Most Foul* (New York, 2018), p. 302.

31 Henrik Schoenefeldt, 'The Historic Ventilation System of the House of Commons, 1840–52: Re-visiting David Boswell Reid's Environmental Legacy', *Antiquaries Journal*, XCVIII (2018), pp. 245–95.

32 Noxious Vapours Abatement Association, Lancashire and Cheshire, November 1876.

33 Peter Brimblecombe, 'Attitudes and Responses Towards Air Pollution in Medieval England', *Journal of the Air Pollution Control Association*, XXVI (1976), pp. 941–5.

34 G. Wang et al., 'Persistent Sulfate Formation From London Fog to Chinese Haze', *Proceedings of the National Academy of Sciences*, CXIII (2016), pp. 13,630–35.

35 Paul D. Blanc et al., 'The Occupational Burden of Nonmalignant Respiratory Diseases. An Official American Thoracic Society and European Respiratory Society Statement', *American Journal of Respiratory and Critical Care Medicine*, CXCIX (2019), pp. 1312–34.

FIVE: LABOURED BREATHING

1 Colin Ogilvie, 'Dyspnoea', *British Medical Journal*, CCLXXXVII (1983), pp. 160–61.

2 M. J. Campbell et al., 'Age Specific Trends in Asthma Mortality in England and Wales, 1983–95: Results of An Observational Study', *British Medical Journal*, CCCXIV (1997), pp. 1439–41.

3 Paul O'Byrne et al., 'Asthma Progression and Mortality: The Role of Inhaled Corticosteroids', *European Respiratory Journal*, CIV (2019), p. 1900491.

4 Sheldon C. Siegel, 'History of Asthma Deaths From Antiquity', *Journal of Allergy and Clinical Immunology*, CXXX (1987), pp. 458–62.

5 Arthur K. Ashbury, 'Guillain-Barré Syndrome: Historical Aspects', *Annals of Neurology*, XXVII (1990) (Suppl): S2–S6.

6   John B. Winer, 'Guillain-Barré Syndrome', *British Medical Journal*, CCCVII (2008), A671.

7   S. Laureys et al., 'The Locked-in Syndrome: What Is It Like to Be Conscious but Paralyzed and Voiceless?', *Progress in Brain Research*, CL (2005) pp. 495–611.

8   A. N. Williams, 'Cerebrovascular Disease in Dumas *The Count of Monte Cristo*', *Journal of the Royal Society of Medicine*, XCVI (2003), pp. 412–14.

9   Stephen W. Littleton and Babak Mokhlesi, 'The Pickwickian Syndrome: Obesity Hypoventilation Syndrome', *Clinics in Chest Medicine*, XXX (2009), pp. 467–78.

10 Peretz Lavie, 'Who Was the First to Use the Term Pickwickian in Connection With Sleepy Patients? History of Sleep Apnoea Syndrome', *Sleep Medicine Reviews*, XII (2008), pp. 5–17.

11 B. Mokhlesi, 'Obesity Hypoventilation Syndrome: A State-of-the-art Review', *Respiratory Care*, LV (2010), pp. 1347–65.

12 Eduardo E. Benarroch, 'Control of the Cardiovascular and Respiratory Systems During Sleep', *Autonomic Neuroscience: Basic and Clinical*, CCXVIII (2019), pp. 54–63.

13 Anon., 'The Black Hole of Calcutta', *The Atheneum*, IX (1821), pp. 278–83.

14 Ronald V. Trubuhovich, 'History of Mouth-to-mouth Rescue Breathing. Part 1', *Critical Care and Resuscitation*, VII (2005), pp. 250–57.

15 Ibid.

16 Ronald V. Trubuhovich, 'History of Mouth-to-mouth Rescue Breathing. Part 2: The 18th Century', *Critical Care and Resuscitation*, VIII (2006), pp. 157–71.

17 Ibid.

18 Ronald V. Trubuhovich, 'History of Mouth-to-mouth Rescue Breathing. Part 3: The 19th to Mid–20th Centuries and "Rediscovery"', *Critical Care and Resuscitation*, IX (2007), pp. 221–37.

19 C.H.M. Woollam, 'The Development of Apparatus for Intermittent Negative Pressure Respiration: (1) 1832–1918', *Anaesthesia*, XXXI (1976), pp. 537–47.

20 Ibid.

21 Arthur S. Slutsky, 'History of Mechanical Ventilation. From Vesalius to Ventilator-induced Lung Injury', *American Journal of Respiratory and Critical Care Medicine*, CXCI (2015), pp. 106–15.

22 C.H.M. Woollam, 'The Development of Apparatus for Intermittent Negative Pressure Respiration: (2) 1919–1976, with Special Reference to the Development and Uses of Cuirass Respirators', *Anaesthesia*, XXXI (1976), pp. 666–85.

23 Leonard Hill, 'Mechanical Respirators', *British Medical Journal*, II/4069 (1938), p. 1389.

24 R. R. Macintosh, 'Mechanical Respirators', *British Medical Journal*, I/4070 (1939), pp. 83–5.

25 Frederick Menzies, 'Mechanical Respirators', *British Medical Journal*, I/4072 (1939), p. 35.

26 Christopher H. M. Wollam, '"A Munificent Gift": Lord Nuffield's Gift of the Both Respirator to the Empire', *History of Anaesthesia Society Proceedings*, XVIII (2015), pp. 105–14.

27 Jeanette Scott and Paul A. Baker, 'How Did the Macintosh Laryngoscope Become So Popular?', *Pediatric Anesthesia*, IXX (2009), (Suppl1): pp. 19–24.

28 Richard Foregger, 'Richard Von Foregger, PhD, 1872–1960. Manufacturer of Anesthesia Equipment', *Anesthesiology*, 84, CXXXIV (1996), pp. 190–200.

29 T.C.R.V. Van Zundert et al., 'Archie Brain: Celebrating 30 Years of Development in Laryngeal Mask Airways', *Anesthesia*, CXVII (2012), pp. 1375–85.

30 Brian W. Rotenberg, Dorian Murariu and Kenny P. Pang, 'Trends in CPAP Adherence over Twenty Years of Data Collection: A Flattened Curve', *Journal of Otolaryngology: Head and Neck Surgery*, XLIII (2016), p. 43.

31 Thomas L. Petty, 'The History of COPD', *International Journal of COPD*, I (2006), pp. 3–14.

32 M. A. Johnson et al., 'Are "Pink Puffers" More Breathless Than "Blue Bloaters"?', *British Medical Journal*, CCLXXXVI/6360 (1983), pp. 179–82.

33 Garry K. Smith, 'Caving for "Pink Puffers" and "Blue Bloaters"', *Proceedings of the Australian Speleological Federation* (2003), p. 11.

34 Robert N. Proctor, 'The History of the Discovery of the Cigarette-Lung Cancer Link: Evidentiary Traditions, Corporate Denial, Global Toll', *Tobacco Control*, XXI (2012), pp. 87–91.

35 Ibid.

36 Ibid.

SIX: BREATHING HIGH AND LOW

1 R. Duffield, B. Dawson and C. Goodman, 'Energy System Contribution to 100-m and 200-m Track Running Events', *Journal of Science and Medicine in Sport*, VII (2004), pp. 302–13.

2 R. Duffield, B. Dawson and C. Goodman, 'Energy System Contribution to 400-m and 800-m Track Running Events', *Journal of Sport Sciences*, XXIII (2005), pp. 299–307.

3 P. B. Gastrin, 'Energy System Interaction and Relative Contribution During Maximal Exercise', *Sports Medicine*, XXXI (2001), pp. 725–41; Valéria L. G. Panissa et al., 'Is Oxygen Uptake Measurement Enough to Estimate Energy Expenditure During High-intensity Intermittent Exercise? Quantification of Anaerobic Contribution by Different Methods', *Frontiers in Physiology*, IX (2018), p. 868.

4 A. V. Hill and H. Lupton, 'The Oxygen Consumption During Running', *Journal of Physiology*, CVI (1922), pp. xxxii–xxxiii; Tudor Hale, 'History of Developments in Sport and Exercise Physiology: A. V. Hill, Maximal Oxygen Uptake, and Oxygen Debt', *Journal of Sports Sciences*, XXVI (2008), pp. 365–400.

5 Gordon C. Douglas, 'A Method for Determining the Total Respiratory Exchange in Man', *Journal of Physiology*, XCII (1911) pp. xvii–xviii.

6 Michael J. Tipton et al., 'The Human Ventilatory Response to Stress: Rate or Depth?', *Journal of Physiology*, DXCV (2017), pp. 5729–52.

7 Ilse Van Diest, 'Interoception, Conditioning, and Fear: The Panic Threesome', *Psychophysiology*, LVI (2019), p. E13421.

8 Colin Ogilvie, 'Dyspnoea', *British Medical Journal*, CCLXXXVII/6386 (1983), pp. 160–61.

9 Van Diest, 'Interoception, Conditioning, and Fear', p. E13421.

10 Ibid.

11 Y. Sakaguchi and E. Aiba, 'Relationship Between Musical Characteristics and Temporal Breathing Pattern in Piano Performance', *Frontiers in Human Neuroscience*, X (2016), p. 381.

12 Andrew B. Lumb, *Nunn's Applied Respiratory Physiology,* 5th edn (Oxford, 2000), p. 685.

13 Cynthia M. Beall et al., 'Hemoglobin Concentration of High-altitude Tibetans and Bolivian Aymara', *American Journal of Physical Anthropology: The Official Publication of the American Association of Physical Anthropologists*, CVI (1998), pp. 385–400; Christina A. Eichstaedt et al., 'Genetic and Phenotypic Differentiation of an Andean Intermediate Altitude Population', *Physiological Reports*, III (2015).

14 Hao Hu et al., 'Evolutionary History of Tibetans Inferred from Whole-genome Sequencing', *PLOS Genetics*, XIII (2017), p. E1006675.

15 Fahu Chen et al., 'A Late Middle Pleistocene Denisovan Mandible from the Tibetan Plateau', *Nature*, DLXIX (2019), pp. 409–12.

16 Sam Kean, *Caesar's Last Breath: Decoding the Secrets of the Air Around Us* (New York, 2017), p. 374.

17 J. B.West, 'Early History of High-altitude Physiology', *Annals of the New York Academy of Sciences*, MCCCLXV (2016), pp. 33–42.

18 Kean, *Caesar's Last Breath*, p. 374.

19 Paul Bert and Fred A. Hitchcock, *Barometric Pressure: Researches in Experimental Physiology* (Columbus, OH, 1943), p. 972.

20 V. Theodore Barnett, 'Respiratory Effects of the Dead Sea: A Historical Note', *Chest*, CXIV (1998), p. 949.

21 M. R. Kramer et al., 'Rehabilitation of Hypoxemic Patients with COPD at Low Altitude at the Dead Sea, the Lowest Place on Earth', *Chest*, CXIII (1998), pp. 571–5; Nedal Alnawaiseh and Fathi El-Gamal, 'The Effect of Low Altitude on the Performance of Lung Function in Alaghwar Region, Dead Sea, Jordan', *Journal of Pulmonary and Respiratory Medicine*, VIII (2018), p. 445.

22 John B. West, 'Snorkel Breathing in the Elephant Explains the Unique Anatomy of Its Pleura', *Respiration Physiology*, CXXVI (2001), pp. 1–8.

23 G. Kim Prisk, 'Microgravity and the Respiratory System', *European Respiratory Journal*, XLV (2014), pp. 1459–71.

24 A. L. Gill and C.N.A. Bell, 'Hyperbaric Oxygen: Its Uses, Mechanisms of Action and Outcomes', *Quarterly Journal of Medicine*, XCVII (2004), pp. 385–95.

25 Carlos D. Scheinkestel et al., 'Where to Now With Carbon Monoxide Poisoning?', *Emergency Medicine*, XVI (2004), pp. 151–4.

26 Chris Acott, 'Oxygen Toxicity: A Brief History of Oxygen in Diving', *SPUMS Journal*, XXIX (1999), pp. 150–55.

SEVEN: BREATHING FAST AND SLOW: BREATHE IN, BREATHE OUT

1 Andrea Zaccaro et al., 'How Breath-control Can Change Your Life: A Systematic Review on Psycho-physiological Correlates of Slow Breathing', *Frontiers in Human Neuroscience*, XII (2018), p. 353.

2 Christopher Gilbert, 'Emotional Sources of Dysfunctional Breathing', *Journal of Bodywork and Movement Therapies*, II (1998), pp. 224–30.

3 Christopher Gilbert, 'Yoga and Breathing', *Journal of Bodywork and Movement Therapies*, III (1999), pp. 44–54.

4 Richard M. Harding and F. John Mills, 'Problems of Altitude. I: Hypoxia and Hyperventilation', *British Medical Journal*, CCLXXXVI (1983), pp. 1408–10.

5 S. Cooper et al., 'Effect of Two Breathing Exercises (Buteyko and Pranayama) in Asthma: A Randomised Controlled Trial', *Thorax*, CVIII (2003), pp. 674–9.

6 Leon Chaitow, Christopher Gilbert and Dinah Bradley, *Recognizing and Treating Breathing Disorders*, 2nd edn (London, 2013), p. 320.

7　Penelope Latey, 'The Pilates Method: History and Philosophy', *Journal of Bodywork and Movement Therapies*, v (2001), pp. 275–82; Penelope Latey, 'Updating the Principles of the Pilates Method – Part 2', *Journal of Bodywork and Movement Therapies*, vi (2002), pp. 94–101.

8　Patricia Huston and Bruce McFarlane, 'Health Benefits of Tai Chi: What Is the Evidence?', *Canadian Family Physician*, cxii (2016), pp. 881–90.

9　Zhen-Xian Zhang, 'Usage of Traditional Chinese Medicine in Treating Intractable Hiccups: A Case Report', *Journal of Integrative Medicine*, xii (2014), pp. 520–23.

10　Joseph S. Alter, 'Modern Medical Yoga: Struggling With a History of Magic, Alchemy and Sex', *Asian Medicine*, i (2005), pp. 119–46.

11　Edgar Williams, *Moon: Nature and Culture* (London, 2014), p. 198.

12　Jon Kabat-Zinn, *Full Catastrophe Living: Using the Wisdom of Your Body and Mind to Face Stress, Pain, and Illness* (New York, 1991), pp. 59–72.

13　Li Changjun et al., 'Effects of Slow Breathing Rate on Heart Rate Variability and Arterial Baroreflex Sensitivity in Essential Hypertension', *Medicine*, xcvii (2018).

14　N. F. Bernardi et al., 'Cardiorespiratory Optimization During Improved Singing and Toning', *Scientific Reports*, vii/8113 (2017), pp. 1–8.

15　Luciano Bernardi et al., 'Effect of Rosary Prayer and Yoga Mantras on Autonomic Cardiovascular Rhythms: Comparative Study', *British Medical Journal*, cccxxiii (2001), pp. 1446–9.

16　Heather Mason et al., 'Cardiovascular and Respiratory Effect of Slow Yogic Breathing in the Yoga Beginner: What Is the Best Approach?', *Evidence-based Complementary and Alternative Medicine*, 743504 (2013), pp. 1–7.

17　Dirk Cysarz et al., 'Oscillations of Heart Rate and Respiration Synchronize During Poetry Recitation', *American Journal of Physiology: Heart and Circulatory Physiology*, cclxxxvii (2004), H579–H587.

18　Hilal Yuksel et al., 'Effectiveness of Breathing Exercises During the Second Stage of Labor on Labor Pain and Duration: A Randomized Controlled Trial', *Journal of Integrative Medicine*, xv (2017), pp. 456–61.

19　Linda C. Pugh et al., 'First Stage Labor Management: An Examination of Patterned Breathing and Fatigue', *Birth*, xxv (1998), pp. 241–5.

20　G. S. Bause, 'Before the Lamaze Method: Bonwill "Rapid Breathing"', *Anesthesiology*, cxxiv (2016), p. 258.

21 Clarence W. Dail, '"Glossopharyngeal Breathing" by Paralyzed Patients', *California Medicine*, cxxv (1951), pp. 217–18.

22 Malin Nygren-Bonnier, Tomas A. Schiffer and Peter Lindholm, 'Acute Effects of Glossopharyngeal Insufflation in People With Cervical Spinal Cord Injury', *Journal of Spinal Cord Medicine*, xli (2018), pp. 85–90; François Maltais, 'Glossopharyngeal Breathing', *American Journal of Respiratory Critical Care Medicine*, clxxxiv (2011), p. 381.

23 Jan-Marino Ramirez and Nathan Baertsch, 'Defining the Rhythmogenic Elements of Mammalian Breathing', *Physiology*, xxxiii (2018), pp. 302–16.

24 Jing Kang, Austin Scholp and Jack J. Jiang, 'A Review of the Physiological Effects and Mechanisms of Singing', *Journal of Voice*, xxxii (2018), pp. 390–95.

25 Ramsey Smith, 'Breathing in Singing', *Journal of Laryngology, Rhinology and Otology*, viii (1894), pp. 305–9.

26 Sauro Salomoni, Wolbert van den Hoorn and Paul Hodges, 'Breathing and Singing: Objective Characterization of Breathing Patterns in Classical Singers', *plos One*, xi (2016), e0155084.

27 Ramsey Smith, 'Breathing in Singing', *Journal of Laryngology, Rhinology and Otology*, viii (1894), pp. 305–9.

28 Rachel B. Goldenberg, 'Singing Lessons for Respiratory Health: A Literature Review', *Journal of Voice*, xxxii (2018), pp. 85–94.

29 L. Bernardi, C. Porta and P. Sleight, 'Cardiovascular, Cerebrovascular, and Respiratory Changes Induced by Different Types of Music in Muscians and Non-musicians: The Importance of Silence', *Heart*, xcii (2006), pp. 445–52.

30 Eugenija Zuskin et al., 'Respiratory Function in Wind Instrument Players', *Medicina Del Lavoro*, c (2009), pp. 133–41.

31 Lia Studer et al., 'Does Trumpet Playing Effect Lung Function? – A Case Control Study', *plos One*, xiv/5 (2019), e0215781.

32 Dietrich Erbert et al., 'Coordination Between Breathing and Mental Grouping of Pianistic Finger Movements', *Perceptual and Motor Skills*, xcv (2002), pp. 339–53.

33 Ramirez and Baertsch, 'Defining the Rhythmogenic Elements of Mammalian Breathing', pp. 302–16.

34 Peter Gilroy, 'A Case of Pulmonary Abscess Caused by the Lodgement of a Chicken Bone in One of the Bronchi', *Edinburgh Medical and Surgical Journal*, xxxv (1831), pp. 293–6.

35 Keith Singletary, 'Oregano: Overview of the Literature on Health Benefits', *Nutrition Today*, xcv (2010), pp. 129–38.

36 www.npg.org.uk/whatson/display/2004/theodore-de-mayerne, accessed 8 November 2020.

37 Poonam Mahendra and Shradha Bisht, '*Ferula asafoetida*:
    Traditional Uses and Pharmacological Activity', *Pharmacognosy
    Reviews*, VI (2012), pp. 141–6.
38 Fred Hageneder, *Yew* (London, 2012), p. 255.
39 Ibid.

EIGHT: INSPIRED BREATHING

1 Corinne Saunders, 'The Play of Breath: Chaucer's Narratives of
   Feeling', in *Reading Breath in Literature* (Basel, 2019), pp. 17–38.
2 Naya Tsentourou, 'Wasting Breath in Hamlet', in *Reading Breath
   in Literature* (Basel, 2019), pp. 39–63.
3 S. O'Mahony, 'A. J. Cronin and The Citadel: Did a Work of Fiction
   Contribute to the Foundation of the NHS?', *Journal of the Royal
   College of Physicians of Edinburgh*, XCII (2012), pp. 172–8.
4 Jean-Thomas Tremblay, 'Breath: Image and Sound, An
   Introduction', *New Review of Film Television Studies*, XVI (2018),
   pp. 93–7.

NINE: LAST GASP

1 Lawrence A. Zeidman, James Stone and Daneil Kondzeilla,
   'New Revelations about Hans Berger, Father of the
   Electroencephalogram (EEG), and His Ties to the Third Reich',
   Journal of Child Neurology, XXIX (2014), pp. 1002–10.
2 Ibid.
3 Calixto Machado et al., 'The Concept of Brain Death Did Not
   Evolve to Benefit Organ Transplants', *Journal of Medical Ethics*,
   XXXIII (2007), pp. 197–200.

FURTHER READING

Arnold, Catherine, *Pandemic 1918: The Story of the Deadliest Influenza in History* (London, 2018)

Braun, Lundy, *Breathing Race into the Machine: The Surprising Career of the Spirometer, from Plantation to Genetics* (Minneapolis, MN, 2014)

Brimblecombe, Peter, *The Big Smoke: A History of Air Pollution in London since Medieval Times* (London, 1987)

Bynum, Helen, *Spitting Blood: The History of Tuberculosis* (Oxford, 2012)

Canfield, Donald E., *Oxygen: A Four Billion Year History* (Princeton, NJ, 2014)

Connor, Steven, *The Matter of Air: Science and Art of the Ethereal* (London, 2010)

Cronin, A. J., *The Citadel* (London, 1937)

Johnson, Steven, *The Invention of Air: An Experiment, a Journey, a New Country and the Amazing Force of Scientific Discovery* (London, 2009)

Kean, Sam, *Caesar's Last Breath: The Epic Story of the Air Around Us* (New York, 2017)

Lougheed, Kathryn, *Catching Breath: The Making and Unmaking of Tuberculosis* (London, 2017)

Pelosi, Paolo, *On the Scent: A Journey through the Science of Smell* (Oxford, 2016)

Smedley, Tim, *Clearing the Air: The Beginning and the End of Air Pollution* (London, 2019)

Süskind, Patrick, *Perfume: The Story of a Murderer* (London, 1985)

West, J. B., ed., *Respiratory Physiology: People and Ideas* (New York, 1996)

ACKNOWLEDGEMENTS

I t has been a great privilege to write this monograph on the history of breathing. This book has allowed me to indulge in my life-long interest in respiratory physiology. When writing papers or lecturing to students, I have often sought the views of earlier researchers, placing their discoveries in context and viewing their contributions and discoveries through a 'modern' lens. Their stories bring history to life. Breathing is a process we all take for granted, but now with air pollution and new infectious diseases it is important that we protect the environment around us, and especially the air we all breathe.

I would like to thank the publishing team at Reaktion Books for all their professional guidance and work needed to produce this book. I wish to thank my family for their support, especially during the long periods of solitary confinement needed to collate the many reports and papers used in supporting and writing this narrative. Karen deserves special mention as the book would not have been written without her constant and unwavering support. The views (and any errors) expressed in this book are all mine and mine alone.

Note: The Covid-19 pandemic was still ongoing when the book was published; it covers events up to the summer of 2020.

PHOTO
ACKNOWLEDGEMENTS

The author and publishers wish to express their thanks to the below sources of illustrative material and/or permission to reproduce it.

Alamy: pp. 124 (Trinity Mirror/Mirrorpix), 171 (World History Archive), 181 (Album), 189 (Science History Images), 190 (Science History Images), 191 (Janie Airey), 201 (ImageBROKER), 229 top right and bottom left (Album); Bridgeman Images: pp. 63 (Photo © Whitford & Hughes, London, UK), 142 (Look and Learn), 176 (Giancarlo Costa); © The Trustees of the British Museum, London: pp. 23 bottom, 100, 101, 205; Centers for Disease Control and Prevention's Public Health Image Library (PHIL): p. 94; Fogg Art Museum, Massachusetts: p. 212; Getty Images: p. 108 (Eric Bouvet); The J. Paul Getty Museum, Los Angeles: p. 130; iStockphoto: p. 114 (hopkinsl); Louvre Museum, Paris: p. 98; The Metropolitan Museum of Art, New York: p. 214; National Gallery of Art, Washington, DC: p. 90; National Museum, Warsaw: p. 111; Shutterstock: pp. 120 (Granger), 146 (Granger), 150 (Everett), 154 (Everett), 169 (Keystone-SDA), 196 (Prostock-studio), 200 (Greg Baker/AP), 216 (Steve Allen); Walters Art Museum, Baltimore: p. 23 top; Wellcome Collection: pp. 36, 39, 47, 67, 80, 85, 117, 156, 157, 160, 227 top left and top right, 231, 232, 234; Wikimedia Commons: pp. 10 (Tate/CC-BY-NC-ND 3.0 Unported), 15 (H. Krisp/CC BY 3.0).

INDEX

Page numbers in *italics* indicate illustrations